# THE BOOK OF
# TOUCH &
# AROMA

# THE BOOK OF
# TOUCH &
# AROMA

*Sensual Ways with Massage
and Aromatherapy*

CYNTHIA BLANCHE

TIME®
LIFE

# Contents

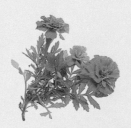

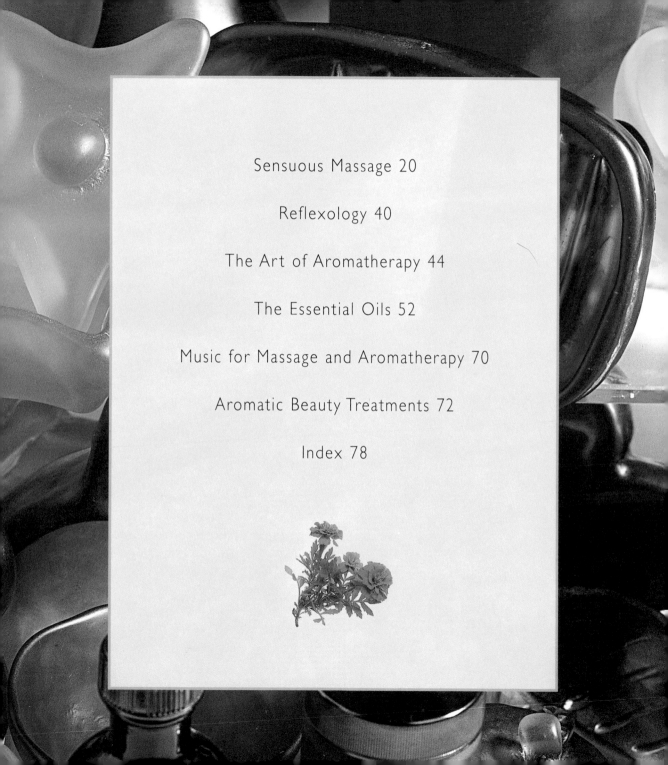

# Introduction

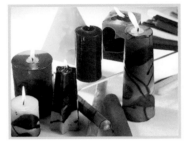

*The more highly attuned our senses, the more we can enjoy life.*
*When we are in touch with our senses, we feel whole as human beings.*
*We can take in the beauty of the world around us.*
*We cherish more fully the people we love.*

When we lose touch with our senses, we may become little more than machines rushing back and forth between work and home, our minds consumed with duties or problems, our bodies forgotten, sensory consciousness mislaid. This is not a desirable or happy state for anyone, yet it is the way many of us live every day of our lives.

We are born sensuous beings. Little children live in their bodies. They are profoundly conscious of every new sensation and experience they encounter in the world. Let your mind drift back to your own childhood. What comes up? Scents and physical sensations most likely — these usually are the most vivid memories we retain from that time before we had to contend with life's stresses.

Have you ever seen a cut on your hand, a cut you couldn't explain? Cuts are painful, but you were too busy to take in the incident — or the pain. And just as you didn't notice the pain of your cut, you are probably not aware of the feel of fabric on your skin, or the scent of the roses in the park you walk through every day, or the aroma of pine needles as they crunch beneath your feet.

Whether or not you are conscious of smell on a day-to-day basis, it is a powerful and important sense and one we should develop and "listen to." We subliminally take in smells all the time. These subliminal odors cause us to feel uncomfortable in particular surroundings and comfortable in others; they cause us to like or dislike a person; they are even largely responsible for choosing with whom we fall in love.

Everyone has a smell that is as distinctive as a fingerprint. Under normal circumstances we are not usually conscious of a person's smell, unless we are in very close physical proximity to him or her — although sometimes we get an exaggerated sense of someone's personal odor when they've been exercising. When we dislike a person on sight, we often think we are being unfair and make an effort to like that person. But it is possible that our instincts, through our olfactory systems, are alerting us to the fact that there is a good reason for our antipathy. The reason could be no more than a simple personality clash — it does not mean that that person is necessarily bad.

The association between smell and emotions is powerful. This is because odors stimulate the same neurons as those used by our emotional center: Most of us have had the experience of walking down a street and becoming conscious of a smell that brings up a vivid memory from the past.

When children meet, they stare at each other for a little while, then begin to play using a lot of body contact. When adults meet — and even when they know each other well — they rarely touch; instead they focus on the organs for speaking, hearing, and seeing. These are the senses our intellects come to rely on, so it is not surprising that as we grow and develop our intellects, we begin to forget to smell the roses in the park and cease to notice the wind on our faces.

Our senses of touch and smell, once reawakened, can have a profound effect on the quality of our lives. They can be the source of great pleasure. If you can recapture a childlike ability to experience every sensation, you will find yourself living in the moment, leaving the past behind, and letting the future take care of itself.

# Becoming a Sensuous Being

*Sensuality reconciles us with the human race. The misanthropy of the old is due in large part to the fading of the magic glow of desire.*

**Eric Hoffer, *Reflections on the Human Condition***

Our bodies are the means through which we experience the world. As children we were acutely conscious of everything that we touched or that touched us and we put everything to our noses to see how it smelled.

When you were small and your parents took you to the beach or to a lake or river, your parents took in the beautiful setting. But you squatted down on the sandy shore and immediately dug your hands into the sand. You wanted to experience the texture of wet sand on your skin and feel the difference between it and the dry sand. You saw the grains of sand before you saw the beach. You were acutely conscious of water rushing around your ankles and the way the sand sank beneath your feet. Every sensation your skin experienced was exciting to you. And so were the smells of the water and the reeds in the shallows of the lake or the seaweed on the beach.

But now you are grown. As adults, the demands of society have taken our minds from the physical sensations of the world to the problems of career and day-to-day living. As we grow up, our minds are concentrated outside our bodies for longer and longer stretches at a time. Then one day, we find that a great chasm between our minds and bodies has developed. We have difficulty experiencing joy. Our relationships suffer through lack of the understanding of one another's needs. We suffer all kinds of stresses that human beings were not genetically designed to deal with.

But this chasm can be removed. The answer lies in rediscovering your senses. Your senses of touch and smell are perhaps the first senses you experienced when you were born. All children are profoundly conscious of them. These senses are potent.

It is difficult to experience the beauty the world has to offer if you are out of touch with your senses of touch and aroma. The ability to see something does not give you the experience of that thing. You need to be able to feel it and smell it to truly experience it. When you see a view you can admire it and walk on. Or you can stand there and close your eyes. Wait a few moments to adjust to your "blindness," then feel the air move, smell the aromas in the air, and sense the vibrations. After a few minutes, open your eyes and truly experience the scene.

Every natural thing in the world has beauty in it. Rediscovering the beauty in the commonplace can be a first step in reconnecting your mind and body. Becoming aware of the senses of touch and smell and learning how to use these senses to enhance your life will make you fully aware of your body and an integrated human being. You will be centered psychologically, your vitality will be increased, and your perceptions will be heightened. The world will become a place of vivid color, of excitement and anticipation.

And once you have a body full of feeling you will be far more sensitive to both your own and your partner's needs. If both you and your partner take this opportunity to reacquaint yourselves with your senses of touch and aroma, those feelings you had when you were first in love will reemerge and a new level of relationship will be forged between you.

# The Importance of Touch

*Touch brings the blind many sweet certainties which our more fortunate fellows miss, because their sense of touch is uncultivated. When they look at things, they put their hands in their pockets. No doubt that is one reason why their knowledge is so often vague, inaccurate and useless.*

**Helen Keller**

Touch is vital for the growth and emotional well-being of people. Children who are raised from birth being cuddled and touched with love grow up to be well-adjusted adults able to establish and maintain healthy relationships. They have high self-esteem and, providing other aspects of their upbringing were nurturing, a healthy sense of their worth to others.

Touch is just as essential in the rest of the animal kingdom. Animals lick their young, not only to keep them clean but to help their development. Birds fuss around their chicks to an extent that might seem overindulgent.

The results of absence of touch have been observed in infants and young children in orphanages where they had little or no physical contact with other people. These children suffered from a condition known as failure to thrive: They were underweight, intellectually underdeveloped, and emotionally distant. Many of them died. But children removed from the situation in time and given constant physical and emotional attention began to thrive. Nursing-home patients who are never or infrequently touched can mentally or emotionally withdraw into deep depression.

Medical studies around the world have shown that massage significantly improves the recovery or health of many patients. Between 30 and 45 minutes a day of massage can prove more effective than drugs in relieving chronic tension and anxiety. The heartbeat of patients whose hands are held improves, even if they are in a coma.

Traditional and tribal cultures tend to have a lot of physical contact with their children for several years after birth. In tribal situations, if the group is to live in harmony, all of its members must have a high degree of emotional stability. Babies are carried by their mothers in slings or pouches and are hugged and cuddled by all members of the group.

The demands of modern society deprive us of much of the physical contact we once had and still need. If we were deprived of sufficient loving touch when we were young, it can be difficult to accept loving touch as adults. Those of us who were not raised under nurturing conditions might have problems with our body image and sense of personal worth. We could be victims of the mind-body split and be fragmented in the way we think and feel. If this sounds like you, be assured that you can reverse this situation.

Massage and aromatherapy are two of the most pleasurable experiences you can have. Using the techniques outlined in this book, you will soon find yourself transformed. Your senses will be heightened, your sense of worth significantly increased. If your body has been a source of humiliation or pain for you, it will become a source of pleasure and harmony.

Our skin is our body's largest organ. It is also the sensory organ that enables us to touch and feel — Mother Nature must be telling us something!

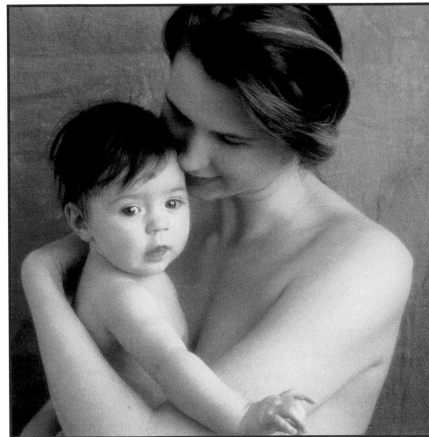

# Connect with Your Body

*Walking barefoot in the park, dancing, feeling the air on your skin,*
*all help to awaken your senses.*

There are many ways that will help you get to know your body that are nonthreatening and fun. They will focus your attention on the feelings of energy flowing within your body and the sensations your skin is registering. These methods are also very relaxing, which is important, because the more relaxed you are, the more in touch with your body you will be. Your body reacts to emotional stresses by tensing up — as if ready to repel an attack.

Whatever activity you do, pausing from time to time to take in and experience the moment will encourage your senses to awaken. If you are walking in the park, for instance, focus your attention on the air on your skin — be conscious of its temperature and whether it is moving or not. Feel it on your face, then your arms and legs, wherever your skin is bare. Feel the wind blow through your hair. Take your shoes off and walk across the grass. Feel the textures, the temperature of the grass beneath your feet. Take in the aromas and try to identify each one.

## Touching Objects

Touching objects with your eyes closed is another way to enhance your sense of touch. Randomly select natural objects, like stones, leaves, and twigs, and pick each one up to fully explore it. Run your fingers over it lightly: Is it cold or warm? Is its texture smooth or rough? Are its edges sharp or blunt? Put it to your nose and smell it.

Don't rush these processes; do them slowly and take in each sensation separately. You will be amazed at how heightened your senses become.

## Looking in the Mirror

After a bath, pat your skin dry with a warm, clean towel — don't rub — and massage some lotion into your skin. As you do this, gaze at yourself naked in the mirror.

This body is the means through which you experience and participate in this world. If you think about your body too much, you will cease to feel through it. Regard your curves and body masses with interest and affection, no matter what shapes they come in, and resist any impulse to criticize yourself.

## Dancing

Dancing is an excellent way of experiencing the energies flowing through your body. It is great fun and allows you to feel the music flowing through your body. It is one of the best antidepressants, and as long as you fully experience it without inhibition, it unites your physical, emotional, and spiritual aspects.

If you feel self-conscious, dance when you are alone. Take the phone off the hook and lock the door. Leave your critical faculties outside and abandon yourself to the music. No one else is there to see if your movements are clumsy, so forget about how you look and allow your body to go with the music. Let all your body parts — feet, legs, hips, bottom, chest, shoulders, arms, hands, fingers, head — be separate entities, entitled to go their own separate ways when the mood strikes them.

Imagine the vibrations of the music entering you — perhaps through your feet from the floor and then flooding upward through your body, or through the solar plexus and radiating throughout your body.

Music that is excellent for getting your whole body moving is traditional Turkish or Arabic music or African tribal music.

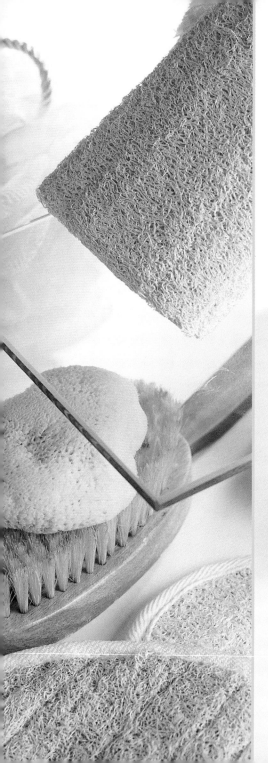

## Dry Loofah Brushing

One of the best ways to begin the process of increasing your body awareness is through light toe-to-top skin stimulation. Before your bath or shower, try stroking a loofah or soft-bristled brush up your body, beginning with your feet.

Make sure the room is warm. Low lighting, especially candlelight, is desirable. Harsh fluorescent lights or lights of high wattage create an oppressive atmosphere that will conflict with your desire to experience the tingling sensation created by the dry loofah. For more ideas on setting the scene, see CREATING ATMOSPHERE on page 16.

Find a position that feels comfortable. You may prefer to stand for the entire process or for just a part. You may prefer to sit or lie down.

The strokes should be light and not too fast — after all, this is supposed to be pleasurable, not something to be over and done with. You can vary the tempo and firmness of the strokes to experience different sensations.

1. Brush the tops of your feet first, from the toes up to the knees in sweeping strokes, all around your lower leg. Stroke beneath your feet from the heel to the toes — if this is ticklish, don't worry, once you become accustomed to it the ticklish feeling will disappear.
2. Next, brush your upper leg from the knees to the thighs. Go all the way around your upper leg in a series of upward strokes toward the heart.
3. Beginning with your left hip, brush the loofah with light, sweeping strokes up toward the heart. Continue making upward strokes, gradually moving across to your right hip with each stroke.

4. Next, brush your back. If standing is difficult for you, find a position that will enable you to do this, e.g., lying on your side, kneeling, crouching, or sitting on a chair. Take the loofah and, in a series of upward strokes beginning from your right hip, brush from beneath your buttocks to your shoulder blades.

5. When you reach your left hip, continue the movement up the inside of your left arm, sweeping across your palm and off your fingertips.

6. Brush the top of your left arm from the fingertips up to your shoulder, then sweep the loofah off your shoulder. Make sure you go all the way around your arm, until you sweep from your fingertips along the inside of your arm and off your armpit.

7. Repeat Step 6 for your right arm.

8. Using very light strokes, run the loofah over your chest and throat area and then, using outward movements, stroke the face, moving from the center toward the ears.

9. To complete the process, put the loofah down and run your fingers through your hair beginning from your hairline, tugging slightly at the ends. When you have completed this process across your entire scalp, take each ear in turn and tug on it gently.

Your skin should be tingling by now. Take a moment to experience this sensation before taking your bath or shower.

When you run your bathwater, put a few drops of an essential oil or a combination of essential oils (see *An Ancient Indian Ritual* on page 49 and THE ESSENTIAL OILS on pages 52 to 69) into the bath. Remember to swish the water well. If you prefer a shower, put some oils onto a loofah or sponge.

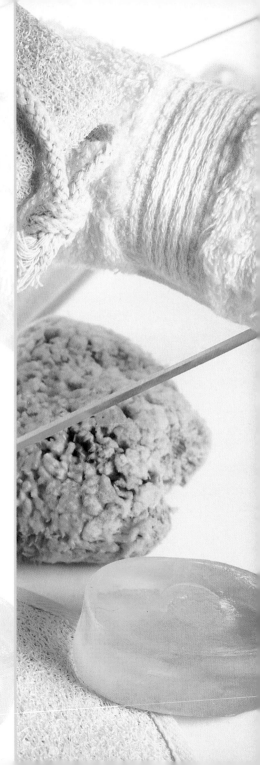

# Creating Atmosphere

*The atmosphere of your environment can have a profound effect on your mood. A cold, dark, dingy room will make even the most impervious person depressed, while a depressed person walking into a beautiful sunny spring garden will immediately feel a surge of joy and well-being.*

No matter how large or small your house or apartment, you can make the atmosphere warm and inviting and, with the use of essential oils, capture something of the ambience of a spring garden.

There is no home whose atmosphere can't be inexpensively improved. If the atmosphere of your home is actually depressing you, you need to stand back and objectively look at each element. For instance, when you look at the color of your walls, does it make you feel happy or gloomy? Colors that make a small room seem smaller will make you feel oppressed. Cool colors in a cold room will make you feel depressed. The biggest expense in repainting a room is hiring a professional to do the work. Do the work yourself, and just by changing the color of the walls, you can go a long way toward feeling happy and energized.

Keeping a room tidy also makes a significant improvement in your mood. Bits and pieces of clothing or junk strewn around will not only clutter up the room but they can make you feel emotionally cluttered as well.

Temperature is also important in creating the right atmosphere. You are tired when you get home from work, so install inexpensive timers on heating or cooling appliances and on lights, so that you can enter a home that seems to be waiting for you.

## *Lighting*

Lighting also influences your emotions. When you are trying to relax, harsh overhead lighting could make you feel oppressed and anxious. The light created by table lamps or candles is soft and relaxing.

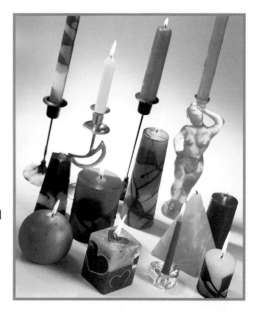

## Table Lamps

Table lamps can be a very attractive asset to a room. Lamp shades are decorative and are available in many styles and fabrics to suit every conceivable purpose and taste. Just changing the lamp shades may be all you need to create a new atmosphere in a room.

## Light Bulbs

Light bulbs can come in many colors. You can buy special paints from craft shops and paint attractive designs on them that will create unusual colors and patterns in the room. You can also dab essential oils onto light bulb rings to suffuse the atmosphere with scent.

## Candles

Candles are very romantic, but a single candle will not produce enough light. These days, you can buy candles of many different styles, shapes, and sizes. Some are steeped in scents designed to lift your spirits, relax you, or encourage romantic feelings. You can put many candles together in decorative bottles if they're narrow and tall, or group them on a low table or on the floor if they're wide at the base — with a little imagination, you can create a spectacular display. You can also buy candelabra to sit on tables or tall stands to place on the floor. A seven-candle candelabrum will produce light equivalent to a 40-watt bulb.

When the candle has burned for a while, put a few drops of essential oils into the melted wax and perfume will suffuse the air.

## Scented Ambience

Research has shown that scent can alter your moods without your even being aware of it. There's nothing like a bowl of aromatic fresh flowers to bring a joyful mood into a room. Another pleasant way to give a room a subtle fragrance is with potpourri. Potpourri is a mixture of dried flower petals and spices kept in an open jar. You can buy the ingredients from florists and craft stores, which you can then put into decorative ceramic containers. Bowls of potpourri are especially attractive in the bathroom.

There are many ways you can use scent to lift your mood. One very easy way is to dab a few drops of your favorite essential oil or up to three different oils onto a handkerchief. When you feel the need, just take it from your pocket or handbag and smell it. This will give you an instant lift and is especially useful if you are feeling depressed, lack energy, or are feeling anxious. For the effects the different oils have on your emotions, see the chart on page 68 or read the descriptions of the various oils in THE ESSENTIAL OILS starting on page 52. You will find that you have an affinity with certain oils and not with others. For instance, if you don't like the scent of an oil, it is not likely to make you feel relaxed and reassured, regardless of its other properties and what it will do for other people.

## Burning Oils

An inexpensive way to fill the air with fragrance is to add a few drops of essential oils to a bowl of water set on a radiator. All you have to do then is to wait for the heat to do its work.

You may prefer to buy an aromatherapy burner. Also known as a fragrancer, aroma lamp, or vaporizer, these attractive ceramic containers have a bowl at the top and an opening at the bottom for a candle. You fill the bowl with water and add up to 8 drops of your favorite essential oils or a combination of oils. The candle creates just the right amount of heat to release the fragrance into the air. It is important to watch the water levels, because if you allow the water to dry out, the oils will leave a sticky residue in the bottom of the bowl.

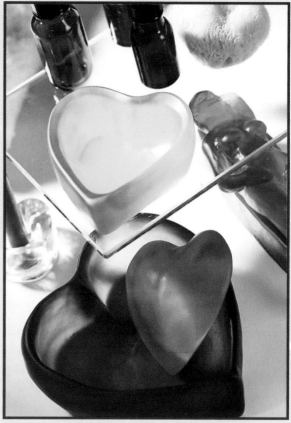

## The Aromabath

One of the most delightful ways to relax and pamper yourself is with an aromabath. Make sure that the temperature of the room is warm enough and that you have plenty of warm, fluffy towels ready to drape yourself in. Roll up one of the towels to use as a headrest while you luxuriate in the warm, but not too hot, water scented with up 6 to 8 drops of essential oils. Add the oils once the bath is full, and make sure you swish the water thoroughly to disperse them.

Candlelight helps create a sensuous ambience as does music playing in the background. Choose music from the list on pages 70 and 71 and you will be in seventh heaven.

An aromabath is something you can share with your partner or someone very special. Use scented bubbles if you prefer, and a glass of champagne would not be out of order.

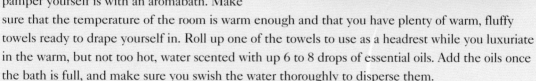

# Sensuous Massage

*Massage can be a relaxing, sensual or euphoric experience, or it can be enlivening, reducing stress and increasing energy. It not only is beneficial to the person receiving it but will calm and restore the giver as well.*

Massage has been practiced as a healing therapy for thousands of years. This should not be surprising, since our first instinct when feeling pain is to rub it away. Archeological digs have revealed that prehistoric humans probably used herbs and potions to rub or massage the body. The ancient writings of China record massage for healing as early as 3000 B.C. Sanskrit writings from 1800 B.C. show massage as a therapy for insomnia, tension, and fatigue. In 5th century B.C., the Greek physician Hippocrates wrote: "The physician must be experienced in many things, but assuredly in rubbing … for rubbing can bind a joint that is loose and loosen a joint that is too rigid." By 300 B.C. the Greeks were commonly using massage with oils for relaxation, beauty, and in the treatment of battle strains and sprains. And the Romans enjoyed massage with scented oils in their private and public baths.

Massage stimulates the skin, the muscles, and blood circulation. It also stimulates the lymphatic drainage system, which is essential to the health of our immune systems. Research has shown that massage releases endorphins — natural hormones that reduce the sensation of pain and increase our sense of emotional, mental, and physical well-being.

Massage encourages openness and gentleness in a relationship. It is a give-and-take experience for both giver and receiver.

## The Techniques of Massage

When massaging someone, you need to be aware of the rhythm, the speed, and the pressure of each stroke or movement you make. These elements will vary according to the stroke and the part of the body to which it is being applied — so watch your partner's reactions. However, strokes that are done at a very slow pace are for relaxation. Increasing the speed will stimulate the circulation to the area, and a brisk movement will warm and invigorate the muscles. The pressure needs to be flexible. You should encourage rather than force muscle to relax. Increase pressure if the muscle seems receptive. Diminish if you feel resistance.

Massage should be a process of flowing movements, each one arising from the last. You can heighten your sense of touch by closing your eyes as you move your hands over the curves and masses of your partner's body.

## Swedish Massage

This is the most common form of massage in the Western world. It generally involves a full-body massage with oils, and incorporates a number of basic massage techniques such as stroking, effleurage, frictions, petrissage, kneading, and percussion (see page 22). Depending on the technique used, a Swedish massage may be relaxing or invigorating. It can be enhanced with the therapeutic use of essential oils.

To enhance the atmosphere, Swedish massage is often accompanied by mood lighting, soothing music, aromas, and hot towels. For more information and some good ideas see CREATING ATMOSPHERE on page 16.

# *The Basic Movements*

### Stroking

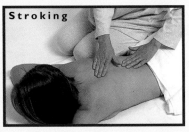
Stroking

The long strokes enable you to make both physical and emotional contact with your partner and locate areas of tension, tightness, or pain. You use long, gentle strokes to spread oil over the area being massaged, using both hands simultaneously or alternating hands. On the arms or legs, stroking is usually in the direction of the feet or hands. Stroking should always be relaxing, soothing, and comforting — use a light touch.

### Effleurage

Effleurage warms the area being massaged and promotes circulation. It also has a relaxing effect on tight, tense muscles. It is generally a long, even stroke applied with firm pressure. It is a movement that has two parts.

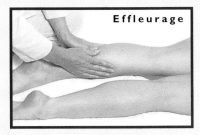
Effleurage

First, slide your hands forward. Usually, both hands work at the same time, either side by side with thumbs touching, or one below the other. On your partner's back, you may move your hands in any direction, but on the limbs your hands should always move in the direction of the heart — this is the opposite of stroking.

Second, after sliding hands forward, lightly draw them back in the opposite direction.

### Petrissage

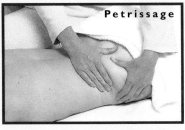
Petrissage

Petrissage helps to relieve muscle fatigue and eliminate the buildup of toxins. It includes a range of movements, such as kneading, rolling, wringing, and squeezing. While stroking and effleurage are long, gliding movements, petrissage concentrates more on specific muscle areas to "soften them up" for deep massage . Petrissage is particularly useful on the fleshy parts of the body.

Kneading in a massage is just like kneading bread. Use each hand alternately to hold and squeeze flesh between your fingers.

# Frictions

Frictions work at a deep level, concentrating on just a small section of the body at one time. This movement is designed to penetrate problem areas of tension buildup.

The pads of your thumbs or fingers are used to make small circular movements. It is also possible to use the heel of your hand. Work slowly and carefully into the area — start gently and increase pressure as you feel the muscle tissue relaxing beneath your fingers.

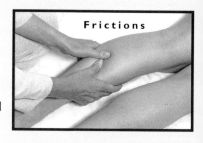
Frictions

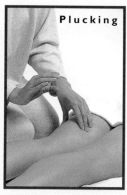
Plucking

# Tapotement

Tapotement, also known as percussion, is made of of brisk, rhythmic movements that are used on fleshy areas of the body to stimulate circulation. The wrists should be loose and flexible, the movements fast and invigorating. Tapotement is good for improving muscle tone and firming sagging skin. Do not use these movements around the kidney area, over the spine, behind the knees, or on any area where there is little flesh between skin and bone. But wherever you use these movements, there should not be any pain.

The movements include:

"Flicking": Using the little finger side of your hands, palms facing each other, hands relaxed and alternately bouncing off the skin.

"Plucking": Pieces of flesh are picked up between thumb and fingers with alternate hands.

"Cupping": Hands and wrists are relaxed with fingers held closely together and arched to form a cup. The cup formed by each hand alternately strikes the skin creating a hollow sound.

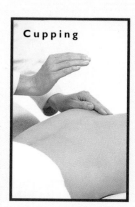
Cupping

"Pummeling": Both hands are held in a loose fist. Using the little finger side, the fists are lightly bounced of the skin, alternating between hands.

Once you have learned and understood these basic movements, try improvising. However, it is important that you try to maintain a rhythmic flow throughout the massage.

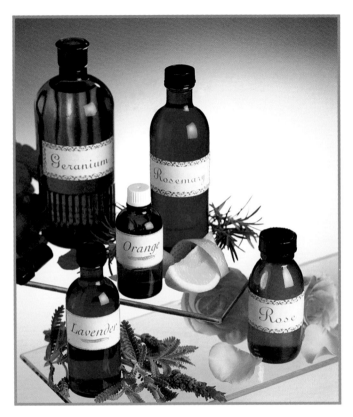

## Using Oils

Massage oils aid the movement of the hands over the skin. They also moisturize and soften the skin. Massage oils can be any good-quality, cold-pressed vegetable oil, though some are preferable to others. When essential oils are mixed into these "carrier oils" and massaged into the skin, their therapeutic properties are introduced into the body. The use of essential oils will greatly enhance the effects of massage, making it a sensuous experience you will want to repeat over and over again.

For a description of most of the most popular essential oils and how they will affect your senses, see THE ESSENTIAL OILS on page 52.

## Carrier Oils

The proportion of essential oil to base carrier oil or water is the most important measurement to remember when making up a blend. Just because a little essential oil is beneficial, it does not mean that a large amount will work better. Use only tiny amounts: The recommended proportions of essential oils to base carrier oils are 12 drops to 5 teaspoons (25 ml) carrier oil for the body; 6 drops to 5 teaspoons (25 ml) carrier oil for the face. Use less for children and women who are pregnant.

The following are popular base carrier oils. You may like to have one or two on hand, since they have different consistencies and will suit you for different purposes.

*Note: All carrier oils should be purchased in dark glass and kept refrigerated once opened.*

**Avocado:** This is a rich and heavy oil that is rarely used on its own, although it is very nourishing and therefore good for dry skin conditions. Add to base carrier oils to help penetration.

**Evening primrose:** This oil is also good for dry skin conditions and can make up 10 percent of a blend with other carrier oils.

**Grapeseed:** This clear, fine oil has no smell and is an excellent carrier oil for massage.

**Hazelnut:** This is a good slightly astringent, penetrating oil. It makes a suitable choice for oily skins.

**Jojoba:** This is not an oil but a liquid wax, so it has the benefit of not turning rancid. Nongreasy and highly penetrative, it softens the skin and hair. Use 100 percent or add to other base oils.

**Olive:** Good as a base carrier oil, this has a strong aroma so it is best used with other base carrier oils. Since this is a warming oil, it is pleasant to use in winter.

**Peach or apricot kernel oil:** Good for mature, sensitive, or dry skin, this finely textured oil is recommended for facial use as it is rich in vitamins and great for cell regeneration.

**Safflower:** This is a good oil for all skin types.

**Sunflower:** This is a good oil for all skin types.

**Sweet almond:** Perhaps the most popular of all and highly recommended, this is an excellent general purpose carrier oil that is neutral, nonallergenic, and good for all skin types.

**Vitamin E:** Mix with base carrier oils such as sweet almond or jojoba to aid penetration of the skin. It is good for facial use and for stretch marks.

**Wheatgerm:** Too rich and heavy to use on its own, this nourishing oil is good for mature skin and dry skin conditions. It is also an antioxidant, so add 10 percent of a total blend to prevent oxidization and rancidity and to provide vitamin E.

# *A Massage Sequence*

## Face and Scalp

1. To begin, have your partner sit upright on the floor, legs outstretched, while you kneel behind him or her. If you find kneeling uncomfortable, sit on a low cushion or soft footstool. Gently lower your partner's head and shoulders, so that his or her head rests against your lower chest. If this is uncomfortable for you or your partner have your partner lie on a towel on the floor.

2. From your chosen recipe, put 4 or 5 drops only on your palms and rub them together so there is no more than a thin film covering your hands. Place your whole hands, tips of the little fingers touching, on the point of the nose. With a light but firm touch, move the tips of your fingers in an arc up from the bridge of the nose and smooth out the forehead to the temples and down toward the cheeks, the rest of your palms moving over the rest of the face. Repeat three times.

3. Place your thumbs together on the center of the forehead and stroke firmly out toward the temples. Repeat three times.

4. Gently knead eyebrows by squeezing and releasing, starting at the bridge of the nose and working all the way to the outer eye, then stroke over the eyebrows with your thumbs.

5. Massage the temple area with the pads of your fingers using small circles in outward movements.

6. Place your fingers under your partner's jaw, your thumbs resting in the hollow of the jawbone. With effleurage strokes, move your thumbs in arcs up the sides of the mouth and nose and out under the cheek bones, continuing the circle under the jawbone. Repeat three times.

7. Place your fingers under the jaw again, your little fingers touching. Pull your hands away from each other, along the sides of the face toward the corners of the eyes. Repeat three times.

8. Using your thumb and fingers, knead the chin area by gently squeezing and releasing. Repeat the movement all along the jaw line to the ears, ending with a soft tug to the ear lobes.

9. Using gentle friction movements with the pads of your fingers, massage around and over the mouth and cheek area.

10. Apply gentle on-off pressure with two fingers at each side of the nostrils, then all the way up under the cheekbones to the temples.

11. Place your hands lightly over your partner's face, little fingers touching. Smooth your hands in an upward and outward arc over your partner's face. Repeat three times.

12. Create frictions with the pads of your fingers over the forehead and then over the entire scalp, always working from the center out. Make sure your touch is firm enough so that the skin moves over the skull.

13. Next, run your fingers through your partner's hair. Lift the hair between your fingers and tug on it gently. Cover the entire scalp.

14. Rub your hands together to create warmth and end by placing your hands over your partner's eyes, your fingers touching between the eyebrows, and hold for about a minute.

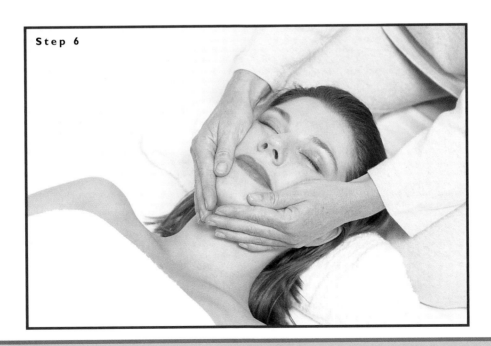

Step 6

## Neck and Shoulders

1. While your partner is still lying on his or her back, pour a small amount of oil into your palm and rub your hands together to create a warm, even slick. Using an even stroke, fan gently from the collarbone out over the chest and shoulders. Repeat 3 times.

2. Cup your hands over your partner's shoulders and stroke up the neck, gently sliding off under the ears. During this movement, apply firm pressure with your thumbs as they travel along first under the shoulder blades, then on either side of the cervical spine (the bones of the neck).

3. Place your partner's head on your knees, making sure he or she is comfortable and relaxed. Take a point on one side of the cervical spine where it meets the skull and make small, deep circles, working all the way along under the ridge of the skull to the ear. Next, work down that side of the cervical spine to the shoulder blade. Repeat small circles moving along a route of outward arcs from the base of the skull to the shoulders until the entire area has been covered.

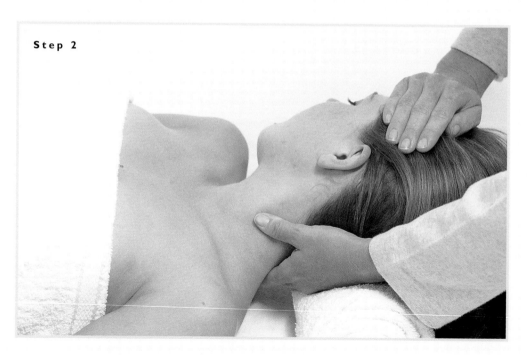

Step 2

Spend more time on any spots that are tight and knotted, but not if it begins to cause pain to your partner. Knots can be worked on gradually over time. Repeat on the other side of the neck.

4. Using the frictions technique, work down to the shoulders, concentrating on the area above and below the collarbone.

5. Cupping your partner's head with both hands, pull gently from the base of the skull and release. *Do not use force.* Repeat 3 times.

6. Finish with long, light strokes from under the ears, down the neck, and over the shoulders and chest area.

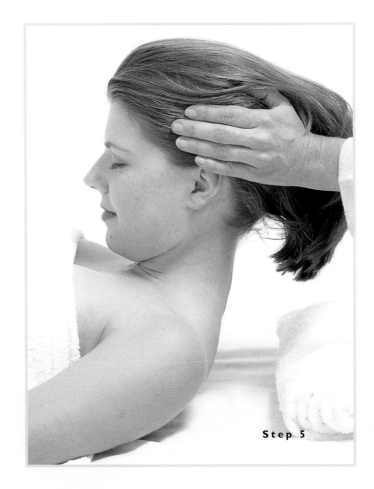

Step 5

# The Chest

1. Your partner should be lying on his or her back. Kneel behind his or her head and pour some oil into your palm. Rub your hands together to warm the oil and create an even slick. Apply the oil by gliding your hands down the middle of your partner's chest. Separate your hands, go around the breast area, and return up the sides of the body.

2. Knead the upper pectoral area — the fleshy area below the collarbone. Squeeze and release the flesh using both hands alternately. Work one side fully, then the other.

3. Using the pads of the fingers and light pressure only, work with friction movements over the breastbone. This area can be quite tender, so keep the pressure light.

4. Move to your partner's side, and using your palms, alternately stroke over the ribs opposite you toward the middle of your partner's body.

5. Repeat on the other side.

6. Cover the chest and shoulders with a towel, and gently press both hands first on the breastbone, then on the pectoral muscles, and release.

**Step 1**

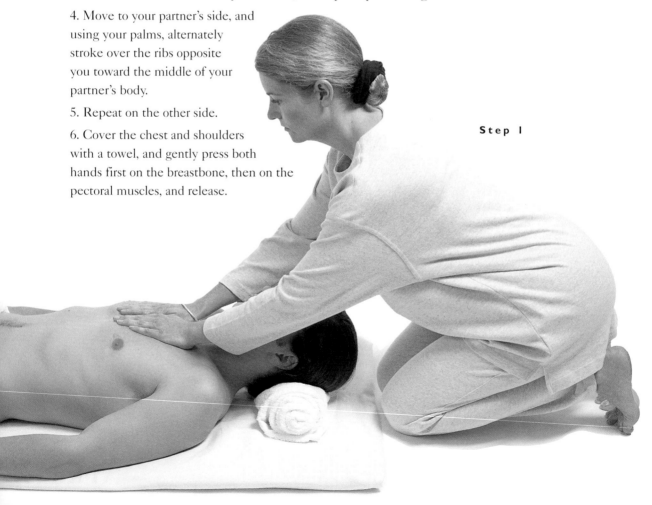

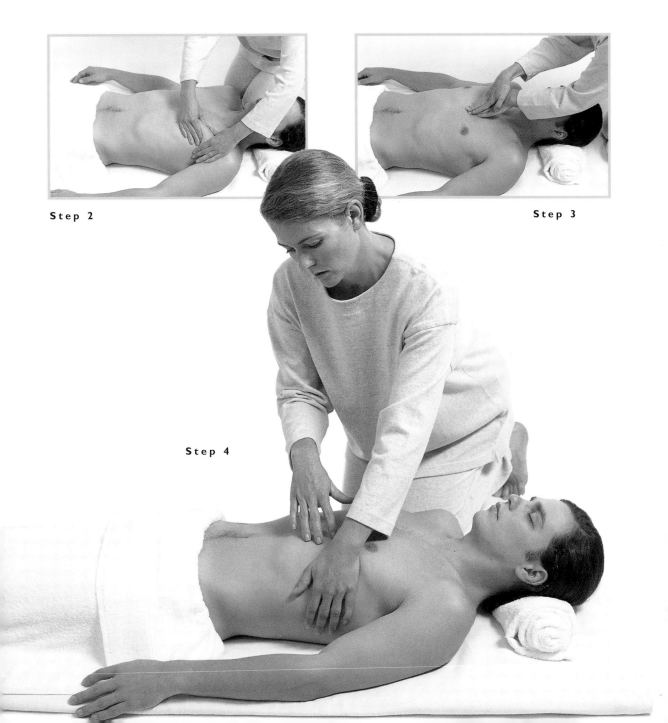

**Step 2**

**Step 3**

**Step 4**

# The Abdomen

1. Kneel on one side of your partner near his or her waist. Apply oil to the whole area with gentle, stroking movements.

2. Effleurage up the middle of the abdomen, out over the lower ribs, and down toward the waist. Pull back down to the lower abdomen, and repeat the whole movement.

3. Gently knead the whole abdomen, starting at the opposite side of the body and working toward you.

4. Using the heel of your right hand, start on the right side of your partner's abdomen and gently push up from the hip area toward the lower rib. Then glide your whole hand across the abdomen, and drag the flat of your fingers down your partner's left-hand side, creating an upside-down U-shape.

5. Gently soothe area with circular effleurage. Your hands should move alternately in wide, clockwise circles, one hand leaving the abdomen as the other makes contact.

6. Follow with a stretching movement. Be sure your partner is relaxed, and execute the movement slowly and carefully — don't pull hard. Lean well over your partner's body. Place one of your hands under each side of your partner's waist. Pull upward, rising onto your knees and straightening your arms. Your partner's waist will lift off the floor, lengthening the whole abdominal region. Let go slowly, allowing your hands to glide across the abdomen and meet in the middle of your partner's body.

7. Repeat gentle kneading to the entire abdomen.

8. Finish with effleurage up the middle of the abdomen, out over the lower ribs, and down to the waist.

9. Cover the area with a towel, and place both your hands on the abdomen, applying gentle pressure, before lifting your hands from the area.

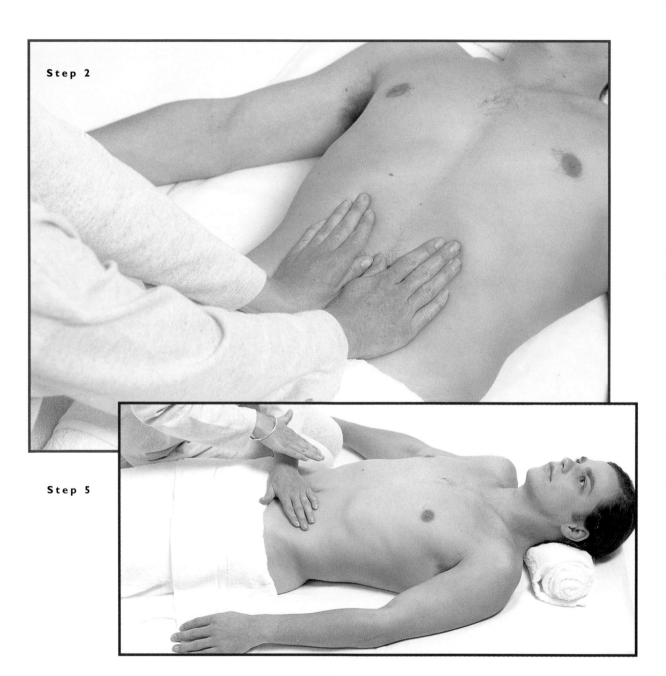

Step 2

Step 5

## Arms and Hands

1. Kneel beside your partner's arm. Pour a small amount of oil into your palm and rub your hands together. Apply the oil to the whole arm with stroking movements.

2. Hold the arm softly at the wrist with one hand, while effleuraging with the other. Glide from the lower arm to upper arm and around the shoulder, and slide back down to the hand.

3. Bend your partner's arm at the elbow and hold the wrist with one hand while the other effleurages toward the elbow and returns to the wrist.

4. Still working on the forearm, try circular friction movements on the area, first on the front and then on the back. Use each thumb alternately to thoroughly massage the whole area.

5. Knead the forearm by sandwiching it between your hands and squeezing in circular movements along the forearm.

6. Rest the forearm across your knee. Now concentrate on effleurage to the upper arm.

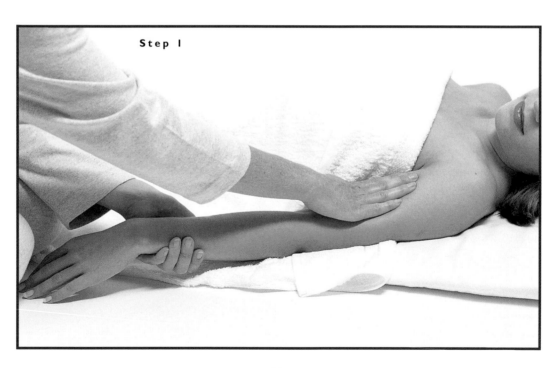

**Step 1**

7. Try friction movements on the upper arm's inner and outer surface along the muscles, using your thumbs and the pads of your fingers.

8. Knead the upper arm by sandwiching it between your hands and squeezing in circular movements up from elbow to shoulder and down again.

9. Move the arm off your knee and effleurage the entire arm to soothe and connect the area.

10. Hold your partner's hand in yours and rub the palm with your thumb. Stroke the upper surface of the hand. Gently rotate the wrist in both directions. Rotate the fingers in both directions and very softly pull them away from the hands.

11. Conclude the arm massage by gently stroking from shoulders to hands. On the final stroke let your hands glide lightly off your partner's. Repeat the process on the other arm.

*Massage of the hands is very reassuring — use your intuition and create your own style.*

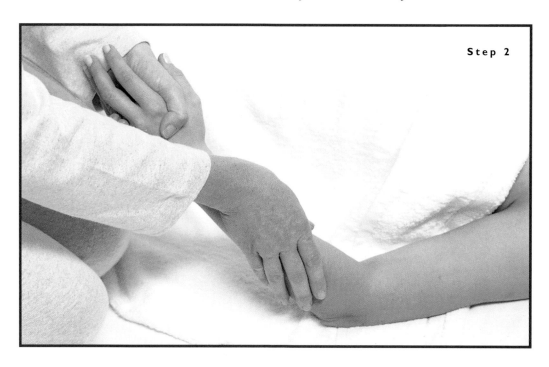

Step 2

# The Back

Your partner should now lie on his or her stomach. Make sure he or she is warm and comfortable.

1. Straddle your partner's thighs and pour a few drops of oil onto your palm. Rub your hands together to warm the oil and create an even slick. Brush your hands lightly, one after the other, down your partner's back as though stroking a cat, gliding off the buttocks. Repeat several times.

2. Repeatedly move your hands up your partner's back from the top of the buttocks in a firm, fanning motion from either side of the spine as though stretching your partner's back away from either side of the spine. As your hands reach the shoulders, press down slightly before gliding around and off the shoulders. Repeat several times.

3. To work the muscles that run along both sides of the spine, use friction movements. Move your thumbs in circles from the base of the spine upward and outward to the top of the spine, then return down the sides of the body in a sweeping stroking movement.

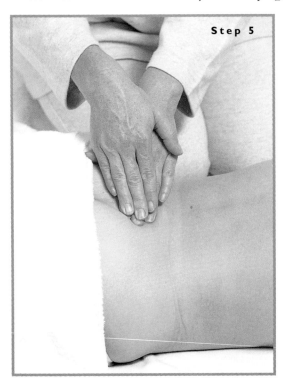

**Step 5**

4. To work the shoulders, knead the upper shoulder muscles. Gently squeeze and release around the entire shoulder area.

5. Move to the side of your partner, kneeling near his or her ribs. You will be massaging the side of the back opposite you. Place both hands on the buttock area, one hand on top of the other. Circle with the hands in wide, sweeping movements from the buttocks toward the head, covering the entire side up to the shoulders. Return, running your fingers lightly down the spine.

6. On the same side of the body, knead the flesh with the heels of your hands. Start at the buttocks with your hands side by side, and push away from the spine with the heels of both hands. Pull back lightly with your fingers, feeling the flesh roll beneath. Work all the way to the shoulders and back to the buttocks with this movement.

7. Knead the buttock area on the side opposite you, using squeezing and releasing movements.

8. Work a little deeper with frictions over the buttocks and base of spine. Use the pads of fingers to locate and work tight muscle areas. Do not press too firmly on the bones at the base of the spine.

9. Move to the other side of your partner and repeat Steps 5 to 8.

10. To finish, move behind your partner's head and brush your hands lightly, one after the other, across the buttocks and up your partner's back, gliding off the shoulder blades.

11. Cover the area with a towel, and place both your hands on your partner's back, applying gentle pressure, before lifting your hands from the area.

*If you like, you may practice some of the tapotement techniques described on page 23. But remember to avoid the kidney area, all bony protrusions, and the spine.*

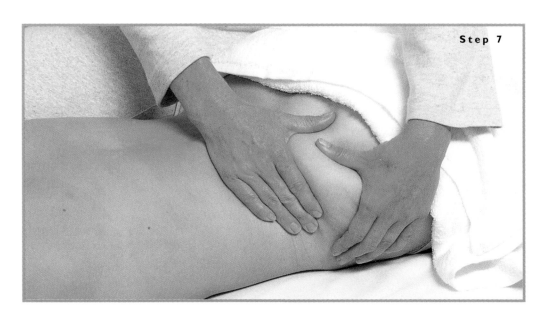

Step 7

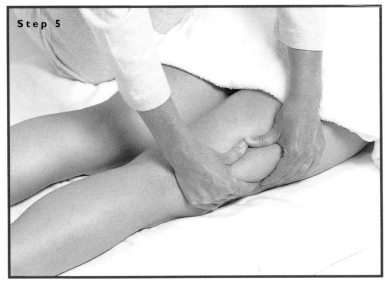

Step 5

## Legs and Feet

1. Kneeling between your partner's feet, apply some oil to your palms and rub them together. Use long stroking movements down the entire leg to the feet to spread the oil. Using effleurage, glide your hands up the leg to the buttocks. With your right hand, curve around the hip and, with both hands, come back down in a long stroke. When you reach the lower leg, slide your left hand under it, your right hand above and continue down the leg, gliding off the feet.

2. Cup your hands. With a firm effleurage movement, push up the calf muscle with one hand — as one hand reaches the top of the calf, the other hand begins with the same movement from the ankle to form a rhythmic, flowing motion.

3. To work more deeply into the muscle mass, use circular thumb frictions. Work up the calf, circling upward and outward. Begin gently, increasing pressure gradually.

4. Move up to the thigh, repeating the same effleurage and friction movements.

5. Kneel by your partner's knee. Knead the flesh from thigh to ankle, then back up to the thigh.

6. Finish with effleurage to the entire leg.

7. To massage your partner's foot, kneel or sit cross-legged near your partner's toes and cradle the foot in one hand. Stroke the foot firmly with the other hand. Begin with firm pressure, as people can be ticklish in this area.

8. Rest the foot on your knee or in your lap and use your thumb in the friction movement to massage in small circles over the entire sole. Alternate between your thumbs.

9. Cup the foot with both hands and effleurage the whole foot with firm movements. Your hands should travel the whole length of the foot.

10. Move to the ankles, circling the ankle bones with the pads of the fingers, and cover the area around and behind the ankles.

11. Work the top of the foot. Support the foot with your hands, and stroke the top of the foot with your thumbs. Glide your thumbs between the small bones of the feet, feeling for the furrows between the bones.

12. Support the foot with one hand on the Achilles tendon (just above the ankle bone at the back of the leg). Rotate the foot first in a clockwise and then in a counterclockwise direction. Do not force the foot if the joint is stiff; work slowly and gently.

13. Rotate each of the toes in both directions. While rotating with one hand, hold the base of the toe with the other hand to add support.

14. Gently pull each toe.

15. Conclude the foot massage with soothing strokes, gently gliding the hands off the ends of the toes.

16. Repeat Steps 1 to 15 with the other leg.

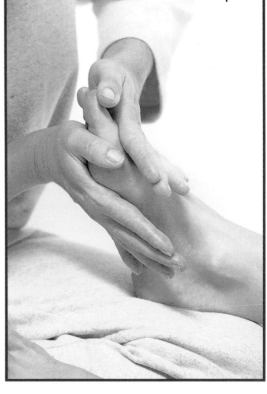

Step 11

*You may like to try some of the tapotement techniques on the back of the legs or pounding techniques on the large thigh muscle. Avoid the area around the back of the knee when using percussive movements. Start very gently.*

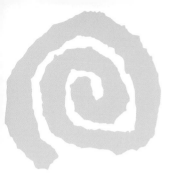

# Reflexology

*Reflexology is based on the concept that a system of
10 energy channels runs vertically through the body, ending
at the feet. The feet are a microcosm of the whole body and
working on particular places on the feet can therefore
stimulate or balance other parts of the body.*

The origins of reflexology can be traced back to ancient Chinese and Egyptian times. In the West, it was developed as a healing art in the early 1900s by an American, William Fitzgerald. Dr. Fitzgerald asserted that all parts of the body are interrelated and that manipulating one part can relieve pain in another part.

Reflexology has been shown to be effective as a relaxation technique and as a reliever of pain as well as stress and tension.

It is easy to learn some of the basic techniques yourself and reflexology can be part of a daily routine. Keep in mind that reflexology is seen as a means to help the body heal itself, not as a cure for any particular problem.

While strict reflexology is difficult to practice on yourself, you can work the different points for 10 seconds or so of on-off pressure. However, it is preferable that you and your partner or a friend swap reflexology sessions. Always work with clean feet and clean hands and make sure the nails of both are short and smooth to avoid scratching your partner. Complete the movements you are going to use on one foot first and then on the other.

# *A Reflexology "Footprint"*

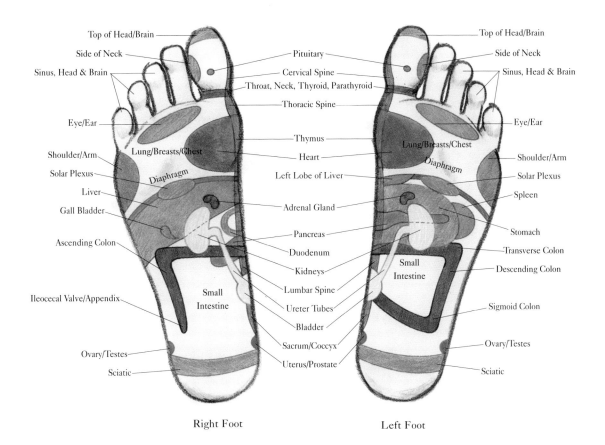

Top of Head/Brain — Side of Neck — Sinus, Head & Brain — Eye/Ear — Shoulder/Arm — Solar Plexus — Liver — Gall Bladder — Ascending Colon — Ileocecal Valve/Appendix — Ovary/Testes — Sciatic — Lung/Breasts/Chest — Diaphragm — Small Intestine

Pituitary — Cervical Spine — Throat, Neck, Thyroid, Parathyroid — Thoracic Spine — Thymus — Heart — Left Lobe of Liver — Adrenal Gland — Pancreas — Duodenum — Kidneys — Lumbar Spine — Ureter Tubes — Bladder — Sacrum/Coccyx — Uterus/Prostate

Top of Head/Brain — Side of Neck — Sinus, Head & Brain — Eye/Ear — Shoulder/Arm — Solar Plexus — Spleen — Stomach — Transverse Colon — Descending Colon — Sigmoid Colon — Ovary/Testes — Sciatic — Lung/Breasts/Chest — Diaphragm — Small Intestine

Right Foot          Left Foot

*A treatment from a qualified reflexologist is a worthwhile opportunity to see the technique in action and to see just how relaxed the rest of your body can feel by working on the feet alone.*

# 10-Step Reflexology Session

1. Cup the ankle in the palm of one hand, and supporting the instep of the foot with the other hand, very slowly and gently rotate the foot around the ankle, first one way and then the other. Move the foot only to the first sign of resistance. Then, slowly and gently, flex and stretch the foot.

2. Next, place your hand around the top of the foot and gently squeeze the base of the big toe toward the base of the little toe — the hollow that results is the first point to use in this session. Release the toes, and using the pad of your thumb, press on this point for a few moments, then begin to make small circles on the point.

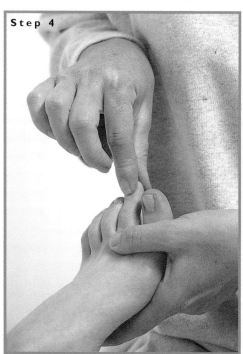

Step 4

3. Hold the feet with both hands your palms on the instep side of the foot. Gently move your hands in opposite directions to "wring" the foot. Move your hands up and down and repeat this movement so that you cover the entire foot.

4. Hold the foot firmly, and with the thumb and index finger of your other hand, massage the whole of the big toe. Then gently rotate the toe, first one way and then the other, and finish by gently stretching the toe. Repeat this step for each toe. The toes correspond to the head and neck, so this is a particularly good area to work if the person is prone to tension headaches and muscular tension around the neck area.

5. Now, make a fist with one hand and use this to support the foot. Using a gentle pressure with the other hand, work from the base of each toe down between the tendons of the foot. Continue to about halfway down the foot.

6. Move one hand to cradle the ankle, and with the other hand still in a fist, use the flat surface created by the back of the fingers to slide from the top of the foot to the ankle. Repeat this two or three times with a firm pressure.

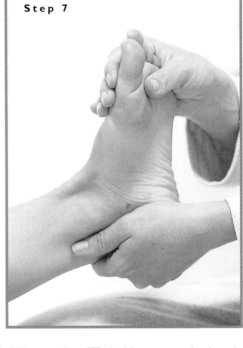

**Step 7**

7. Hold the ankle of the foot to support it and then, using the side of your thumb with short strokes, "walk" your thumb over the ball of the foot. The ball of the foot represents the lungs and chest area.

8. Keeping your supporting hand around the instep, use the other hand to work small circular movements all around the ankle and Achilles tendon. Work this area gently since it can be quite tender on a stressed person.

9. Now, using the pad of your thumb, move with firm circles over the edge and pad of the heel. This area corresponds to your lower back.

10. Finish the session by stroking the foot with the flat of your hand, from ankle to toes and then from the instep to the toes.

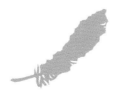

# The Art of Aromatherapy

*Scent can alter your emotions. Unpleasant smells can adversely affect your emotions and you can become anxious and irritable. And if you are feeling low, then the right scent can lighten your mood.*

## The Power of Scent

Animals use their sense of smell to safeguard their lives. Smell, more than sight or sound, warns them of danger from stealthy predators or poisonous substances. Human beings also have this sense, but as our brain power increased over the ages, we began to listen to our intellects rather than our sense of smell when it came to matters of health and safety. Even when we sense that something or someone is wrong, we will dismiss our feelings. Ignoring our gut instincts can lead to fatal errors of judgment.

Through our sense of smell, we can actually detect molecules in the air and distinguish among them with greater sensitivity than any machine. Of course, all this happens on a subliminal level, which is why we often dismiss the significance of our sense of smell.

Smell is perhaps the strongest stimulant of memory there is. If you detect a smell that has an association with something from your

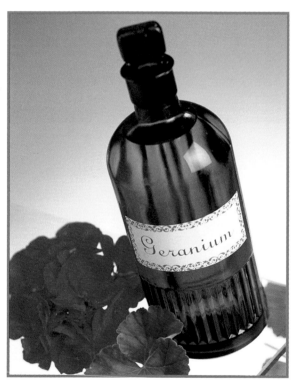

childhood, a full and vivid memory of that event will come to you. The reason for this is that odors and emotions are processed by neurons in the same area of the brain.

Our sense of smell is so important, it can even tell us who our ideal mates are. And there is nothing quite like the joy we experience when the scent of a favorite flower unexpectedly wafts into our noses.

## A Living Essence

An essential oil is a highly concentrated extract from a part of a plant — leaves, petals, bark, seeds, stalks, and flowers — and is indeed the living essence of the plant.

## Aromatherapy

Aromatherapy is the therapeutic use of essential oils to help balance the mind and body. Records of the therapeutic use of oils date back thousands of years to the ancient Egyptians, Indians, and to the ancient Chinese, who believed "a perfume is always a medicine." The Greeks learned from the Egyptians and used essential oils in their baths and massages. Hippocrates prescribed aromatic baths and scented massages using certain oils for protection against contagious diseases.

The Romans reveled in the sensuousness of scented baths and massages. They used them as well to heighten the pleasure of social occasions. Scented ointments were rubbed on the feet of the guests at banquets. Nero imported the costliest of dried Persian roses, walking and sleeping on their petals. He ordered that rose water be sprayed through the rooms of his banqueting hall to perfume his guests.

In the Middle Ages, monks cultivated herbs and discovered many of their restorative properties. They were among the first to distill plant essences, carefully blending them into liqueurs to be administered to patients.

Aromatherapy is not limited to the sense of smell. The essential properties of the oil can also be absorbed through the hair follicles on the skin. These properties are then transported around the body and affect various organs and body systems.

Aromatherapists can choose from about 300 essential oils that are now traded around the world. For home use, you would normally need no more than 30 of the most common and readily available oils and 10 to 12 oils should be sufficient for all the requirements of the average household.

# Aromatherapy in Ancient Egypt

Essential oils were so highly prized in ancient Egypt that tomb robbers would scrape out any remaining ointment with their fingers after emptying the jars of their contents. Unguents, oils, and perfumes were routinely sealed in the tombs of royalty and the nobility.

Egypt's climate was then, as it is now, hot, dry, and dusty. This had a devastating effect on the skins of the people. The poor washed in canals or ponds alive with organisms and larvae that further damaged their skins.

The rich, however, bathed in scented water in luxurious bathrooms. Servants massaged perfumed oils into their skins to stop dryness and to maintain the suppleness and sensuality of youth. Pregnant women had special oil-based unguents that they, or their servants, massaged into their skins to prevent stretch marks. These oils were stored in jars shaped like a naked, pregnant woman holding her belly.

The oils were likely to have been balanos, safflower, linseed, ben, olive, almond, and sesame. Fat from the hippopotamus, crocodile, and cat were also used as massage lotions. The perfumes were produced by steeping various substances in oil: the flowers of the white lily (the Madonna lily), slivers of coniferous timber, fragrant barks, resins like myrrh and frankincense, and sweet-smelling grasses and herbs.

The ancient Egyptians were extremely beauty conscious and used cosmetics extensively. There are many surviving depictions in wall paintings of women applying cosmetics using a mirror (mirrors were, like the oils, perfumes, and cosmetics, regarded as essential equipment in keeping the deceased one beautiful in the afterlife).

The *Ebers Medical Papyrus* suggests: *To remove facial wrinkles: frankincense gum, wax, fresh balanites oil and rush-nut should be finely ground and applied to the face every day. Make it and you will see!*

## Frankincense and Myrrh

Frankincense and myrrh were so precious that they were on a par with gold. These, along with gold, were the greatest gifts the three wise men could bring Jesus. The constant references throughout the Bible to God anointing his people with holy oils composed of frankincense and myrrh show how precious the oils were to the people of Israel. And they were just as precious as religious oils to the Egyptians and the rest of the ancient world. It was unthinkable not to include frankincense in a royal tomb.

> *Place myrrh upon your head,*
> *dress yourself in the finest of linens.*
> **New Kingdom poem**

Wigs were worn by both men and women in Egypt of the New Kingdom. They were believed to increase the wearer's sexual attractiveness. Wall paintings showing the nobility at play have revealed an addition to the wigs, no doubt intended to further increase the owner's sensuality. High cones are perched on the crown of each wig. These cones were believed to be made from animal fats impregnated with myrrh. As the temperature grew warmer at the banquet, the cones would melt and run down the wig and clothing of the guest, leaving them fragrant and cool. Servants would be busy topping up the cones as they melted. In the wall paintings, the cones are shown as white lumps with brown streaks running down the sides. White clothing worn by the guests is stained by brown marks at the shoulders.

Frankincense is regarded by modern-day aromatherapists as one of the most luxurious oils for treating mature skin. Frankincense and myrrh are capable of bringing out all that is sensual in us; they are, as well, still used in religious rituals to create a bridge between heaven and earth.

## *Sensual Rituals*

Most ancient civilizations had many rituals to celebrate sensuality, sexuality, and spirituality. The ritual on the page opposite is an adaptation of an ancient Indian ritual.

By using the senses of touch and aroma, you can create your own rituals to enhance your relationship. While these are wonderful ways to heighten an already harmonious relationship, rituals are especially useful if your relationship is suffering from problems of communication. Loving touch is nurturing, and scents can open the heart and help break down defensive barriers.

Scents affect different people differently, so it is important you and your partner take the time to discover which oils you find most sensual. And remember that essential oils should always be used in small quantities, no matter what the purpose. In the case of a sensual scent, instead of heightening your senses, too much will nauseate you and become anaphrodisiac.

### Aphrodisiac Oils
Anise • Basil • Bergamot • Black pepper
• Clary sage • Fennel • Frankincense
• Geranium • Ginger • Jasmine • Juniper
• Lime • Myrrh • Orange • Patchouli • Rose
• Sandalwood • Vetiver • Ylang-Ylang

## An Ancient Indian Ritual

The Rite of the Five Essentials is part of the preparatory stage of one of the rituals known as *Maithuna*, which comes from the ancient Indian school of tantric yoga. In tantric yoga, a man and a woman, representing the universal male and female polarities, worship each other.

In the Rite of the Five Essentials, the man — representing the god, Shiva — is instructed to anoint the body of the woman — representing the goddess, Shakti — with precious oils while uttering certain sacred sounds or mantras. This invokes the goddess energy within each part of the woman.

The ritual of *Maithuna* is sacred and secret; however, you and your partner can perform this part of the rite. To take full advantage of its beauty, first create a tantalizing atmosphere. Remove any clutter from the room and ensure it is warm. Decorate the space with flowers and light some candles — their warm glow will soften the atmosphere, helping the flow of love and communication between you.

*Stroke the woman's hands with jasmine*
*Apply patchouli to her neck and cheeks*
*To her breasts, musk*
*Comb spikenard into her hair*
*Anoint her thighs with sandalwood.*

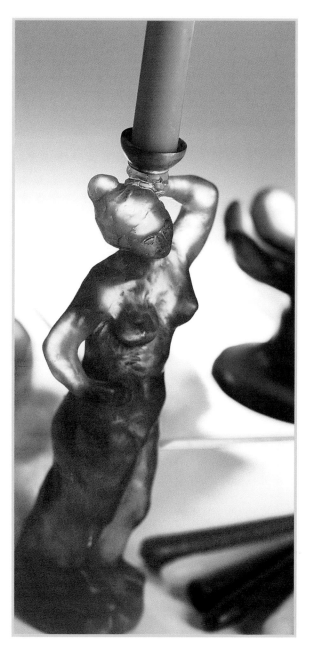

## Precautions

Essential oils are very strong and, with the exception of lavender, should not be applied to the skin undiluted. Even when diluted, some oils may cause an allergic reaction in some people, however, so do a patch test with each essential oil to ensure that you are not allergic to it. If you react with itchiness, blistering, or any other allergic reaction, do not use this essential oil.

While most oils are safe to use, some (including basil, cedarwood, clary sage, ginger, hyssop, juniper, marjoram, pennyroyal, sage, and thyme) should be avoided during pregnancy. Other oils, such as the citrus oils and lemongrass, are phototoxic and should not be used on the skin if it will be exposed to sunlight.

If you are unsure of the use of any oil, are prone to allergic reactions, or are pregnant, or if you suffer from high blood pressure, epilepsy, or another neural disorder, it is best to consult a professional aromatherapist or medical practitioner before using aromatherapy.

## About "Notes"

Scents, like music, have notes. And like music, scents have been regarded as bridges to heaven — hence their use for thousands of years in religious rituals.

The concept of "notes" is one used in perfumery and aromatherapy. A good blend of essential oils often combines all three notes: The top note gives the initial scent and quickly evaporates. In aromatherapy, these are the most stimulating and uplifting oils. The middle note lasts longer and affects your metabolism and body functions. The base note is slower to evaporate, lasting for days, and are the most sedating and relaxing oils. Some oils can act as top and middle or as middle and base notes.

**Top-note oils:** Anise, basil, bergamot, clary sage, eucalyptus, fennel, ginger, grapefruit, lemon, lemongrass, lime, orange, palmarosa, peppermint, petitgrain, Scots pine, rosewood, sage, tea tree, thyme

**Middle-note oils:** Anise, black pepper, chamomile, clary sage, cypress, fennel, geranium, jasmine, juniper, lavender, marjoram, neroli, orange, peppermint, petitgrain, pine, rose, rosemary, rosewood, thyme, ylang-ylang.

**Base-note oils:** Benzoin, cedarwood, cypress, frankincense, jasmine, myrrh, neroli, patchouli, rose, sandalwood, vetiver, ylang-ylang.

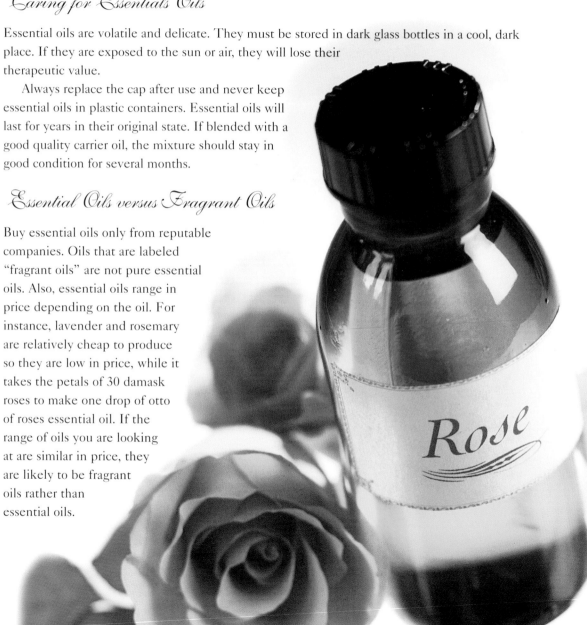

## Caring for Essentials Oils

Essential oils are volatile and delicate. They must be stored in dark glass bottles in a cool, dark place. If they are exposed to the sun or air, they will lose their therapeutic value.

Always replace the cap after use and never keep essential oils in plastic containers. Essential oils will last for years in their original state. If blended with a good quality carrier oil, the mixture should stay in good condition for several months.

## Essential Oils versus Fragrant Oils

Buy essential oils only from reputable companies. Oils that are labeled "fragrant oils" are not pure essential oils. Also, essential oils range in price depending on the oil. For instance, lavender and rosemary are relatively cheap to produce so they are low in price, while it takes the petals of 30 damask roses to make one drop of otto of roses essential oil. If the range of oils you are looking at are similar in price, they are likely to be fragrant oils rather than essential oils.

# The Essential Oils

## Basil  *(Ocimum basilicum)* • Herb • Top Note

The sweet, anise aroma of this oil awakens and arouses the senses. Originally from India, basil is now grown around the world and is used extensively in Mediterranean, Indian, and Asian cuisines.

Basil calms the stress caused by anticipation or anxiety. It has an uplifting, clarifying effect on the brain and may even revive interest in a waning relationship.

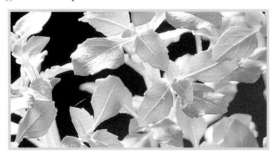

A strengthening oil, basil aids concentration and the processes of decision making. It is an excellent nerve tonic and relieves mental fatigue.

For relief of migraine, headaches, and head colds, use in a steam inhalation, oil burner, or in a massage-oil blend. Use in a massage-oil blend for aching muscles.

*Caution: Do not use during pregnancy.*

## Bergamot  *(Citrus bergamia)* • Fruit Rind • Top Note

Bergamot's fresh, citrusy aroma lifts the spirit and creates a sensual ambience, especially when blended with aphrodisiac oils. It is often used in perfumes and is what gives Earl Grey tea its distinctive flavor. The oil is pressed from the fresh rind of a miniature orange from the Northern Italian town of Bergamo.

It is especially reviving before a night out. It alleviates tension and anxiety, so it is useful when you are feeling distressed or anxious.

Though bergamot is especially good in a facial oil for oily skin or skin that reacts to stress, it suits most skin types. It provides temporary relief from the symptoms of acne, cold sores, eczema, and dermatitis.

*Caution: May be irritating to sensitive skin and may increase skin photosensitivity. Do not use before exposure to sun.*

## Black Pepper *(Piper nigrum)* • Berry • Middle Note

This warming, penetrating, and strengthening oil is distilled from the berries of a vine that grows in India, Indonesia, and Brazil. The aroma of this oil emits the heat of the sun and warms the emotions as well as the body, adding zest to your love life. Its reputation as an aphrodisiac is thousands of years old.

The oil of black pepper was highly valued by the ancient Arabs as an aid to problems of a sexual nature and by the Romans as a physical and sexual stimulant. The Indians and the Chinese used black pepper oil to stimulate the healing process.

Tense, stiff muscles, rheumatism, and arthritis benefit from a massage blend of black pepper oil. Used in an aromatherapy burner, it clears the mind and stimulates energy levels.

*Caution: Use externally only. Excessive use may irritate the kidneys. Do not use during pregnancy.*

## Calendula *(Calendula officinalis)* • Flower

An herb to "comfort the heart and spirits," so say the ancients. The essential oil of calendula, or the common marigold, can help you gain harmony and unity within yourself or your relationship. It is especially useful if there are problems in your relationship that are causing hostility or defensive behavior. Use in a massage-oil blend to calm and soothe your spirits.

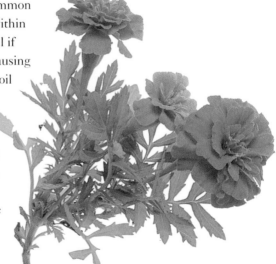

Its soothing qualities are ideal in a skin or facial oil for sensitive skins. Work-damaged hands or skin that has been exposed to chemicals or extremes of temperature will also benefit from calendula oil. Calendula is well known as an ointment effective in the prevention of scars. Use direct application when treating wounds or damaged skin.

## Cedarwood *(Cedrus atlantica)* • **Wood** • **Base Note**

From ancient times, the cedar tree has often been associated with fertility. Known in many parts of the world as the Tree of Life, it has been regarded as a symbol of religious and spiritual strength and as such is used in religious ceremonies.

The scent of cedarwood oil is calming and reassuring and helps in opening up the emotions. When spending time with someone special, cedarwood will help you and your partner live in the moment. Use in a therapeutic bath or burn some cedarwood oil in an aromatherapy burner. Cedarwood is also beneficial in a massage-oil blend.

As a skin-care aid, it has been valued since ancient times as a preserver of youth. It is especially suitable for oily skin. Cedarwood oil is a popular ingredient in men's toiletries.

When used in a steam inhalation or a therapeutic bath, cedarwood oil brings temporary relief to bronchial cough, congestion, sinusitis, and the symptoms of catarrh.

*Caution: Do not use during pregnancy.*

## Chamomile *(Anthemis nobilis)* • **Flower** • **Middle Note**

Also known as Roman Chamomile, this soothing oil has a scent that is invaluable in balancing sensitive emotions. Its nonallergenic properties make it a perfect skin or facial oil for delicate or sensitive skin and has been used for centuries to treat dermatitis, eczema, and skin inflammation. Use in a massage-oil blend or in an aromatherapy burner or therapeutic bath for the temporary relief of headache, migraine, the symptoms of insomnia, and the effects of stress and tension.

Blue Chamomile or German Chamomile (*Matricaria chamomilla*) is excellent for inflammatory skin conditions.

*Caution: Should not be used in the early months of pregnancy.*

## Clary Sage *(Salvia sclarea)* • Herb • Top to Middle Note

Regarded as the most euphoric of all the essential oils, clary sage helps release inhibitions and boost libido, especially when you are under stress. It is frequently used in blends to enhance lovemaking.

Clary sage's relaxing and calming yet intoxicating properties are believed to help release emotional blockages, strengthening one's ability to trust in another. This oil is especially beneficial to depressed people or people who have difficulty letting go and having a good time. Use in an aromatherapy burner, in a therapeutic bath, or for massage.

Clary sage is useful in a massage blend for relaxation, and for the relief of menstrual pains and premenstrual stress. It also gives temporary relief from headaches.

*Caution: May cause drowsiness. Do not combine with alcohol or use before driving. Not to be used by persons suffering from epilepsy. Avoid use during pregnancy.*

## Cypress *(Cupressus sempervirens)* • Leaf & Berry • Middle to Top Note

This oil was so highly prized by the Egyptians for its preservative properties that they devoted it to their pharoahs. Used in a facial-oil blend with neroli and geranium, it treats broken capillaries, tones and refines oily skin, and tightens enlarged pores.

A highly astringent oil, cypress is invaluable for those suffering from fluid retention. Use in a massage-oil blend. Massaging with a cypress-oil blend will nourish veins and arteries and work on the peripheral circulation to relieve aching limbs. Its drying properties and strong, smoky aroma make it an excellent deodorant and men's aftershave.

*Caution: Avoid use if you suffer from high blood pressure. Do not use during pregnancy.*

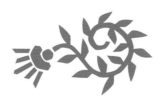

**Frankincense** *(Boswellia carteri)* • **Resin** • **Base Note**

Distilled from the resinous gum of a small tree in the Middle East, frankincense was one of the ancient world's most prized substances. Its aroma is haunting and evocative, one to which you can become quite addicted. Known for its ability to expand consciousness, it has been used from time immemorial for spiritual and religious purposes.

Frankincense opens up communication between people. It calms the mind and stimulates the senses. If you are feeling a little disordered, frankincense will help integrate your emotions. Use it in an aromatherapy burner or bath when suffering stress or when you just wish to enjoy the relaxation that frankincense brings.

In ancient Egypt, frankincense was used in cosmetics to rejuvenate mature skin. Use in skin- and facial-oil blends to protect and strengthen mature skin.

Frankincense also gives temporary relief from the symptoms of bronchial problems and catarrh.

**Geranium** *(Pelargonium graveleons)* • **Herb** • **Middle Note**

The value of this oil is in its ability to create balance. It has a balancing effect on the mind and the body as well as on relationships. Its scent is a mixture of rose and mint and is very refreshing, uplifting, and centering.

To bring balance to a stormy relationship or one in which there are unresolved issues, try the calming effects of geranium in an aromatherapy burner or use it in a massage-oil blend. It will aid communication and help dispel defensive feelings.

Geranium oil is equally balancing to the skin. Use in a skin or facial blend for skin that is either too dry or too oily. It will nourish mature skin, bringing to it a healthy glow.

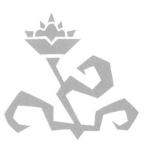

**G i n g e r** *(Zingiber officinalis)* • **R h i z o m e** • **T o p  N o t e**

This oil has had a reputation as an aphrodisiac since ancient times. The Romans used it and so did the Turks. Ginger warms and invigorates the senses and the body.

When used as an inhalation, in an aromatherapy burner, or massage-oil blend, its warming and drying properties give temporary relief to colds and flu and the symptoms of catarrh. It is also comforting to use in a massage oil blend for rheumatic conditions, muscular aches, and stiff joints. Ginger also helps indigestion and nausea.

*Caution: This oil may be irritating to sensitive skin. Do not use during pregnancy.*

**J a s m i n e** *(Jasminium officinalis)* • **F l o w e r**
• **M i d d l e  t o  B a s e  N o t e**

This is one of the most expensive of the essential oils, but it is also among those that last the longest. Jasmine originated in Asia, where it was considered sacred. It has a long history as a flower of love and is a common ingredient in love spells and potions. The heady scent of jasmine is seductive to both men and women.

The aroma of jasmine cannot help but imbue you with confidence, so it is a good oil to use in your bath or as a massage blend before a big date. Jasmine is conducive to love, so use it in a massage blend to share with your partner. Because of its expense, jasmine is usually sold 3 percent essence in a jojoba oil base — this makes it unsuitable for burning in an aromatherapy burner.

A few drops of jasmine in a facial-oil blend will do wonders for dry or mature skins.

*Caution: This oil is not to be used during pregnancy, but is considered to be a useful oil to use during childbirth.*

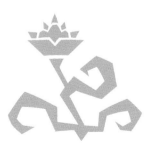

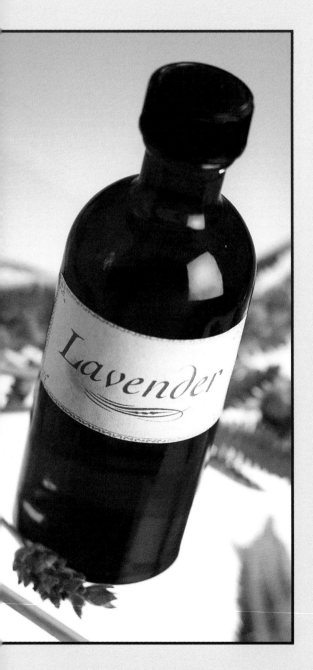

## Juniper *(Juniperus communis)* • Berry • Middle Note

Juniper oil has stimulating and cleansing properties, both emotionally and physically. On the emotional level, it helps you rid the mind of negativity and old bitterness that might be standing in the way of a successful relationship. Juniper has a long history as a protector against negative forces. Use it in an aromatherapy burner or in a massage-oil blend if you are feeling insecure in love or if you need to feel protected. Juniper also gives you strength and resolve.

Juniper helps cleanse the body of toxins. It acts on fluid retention and will help relieve premenstrual swelling and swollen feet.

Juniper's wood-spice aroma and stimulating properties make it an ideal ingredient in men's aftershave.

*Caution: Do not use during pregnancy. Excessive use may irritate the kidneys.*

## Lavender *(Lavendula officinalis)* • Flower • Middle Note

A very evocative scent and soothing to the heart and mind, lavender is perhaps the most popular of all the oils. It blends well with other oils and because of its balancing, comforting, and nurturing qualities, is often included in recipes for lovemaking and the healing of rifts.

Lavender encourages sleep and brings relief to stress and tension. It is an excellent oil to rub onto the temples and neck for relief of headaches, and it is so gentle, you can apply it neat. Use it in an aromatherapy burner, in a massage-oil blend, or put a few drops on your pillow at night.

An excellent oil to use in a facial blend for sensitive and skin that reacts to stress, lavender soothes the inflammation caused by eczema and psoriasis.

## Lemon *(Citrus limonum)* • Fruit Rind • Top Note

With its brilliant, sun-filled aroma, lemon uplifts the emotions. It relieves fatigue and increases mental clarity and alertness. Lemon adds vitality and a sense of fun and abandon to time spent with your partner. If you are about to go out on a big date, lemon will settle your nerves and fill you with optimism. Use in an aromatherapy burner, in a bath, or in a massage-oil blend.

As part of a skin-care oil blend, lemon will brighten pale and dull complexions. It is especially useful for oily complexions.

For relief on a hot day, use a compress soaked in water dispersed with a few drops of lemon.

*Caution: May be irritating to sensitive skin and may increase photosensitivity. Do not use before exposure to the sun.*

## Lemongrass *(Cymbopogan citratus)* • Leaf • Top Note

Lemongrass has a wonderful uplifting scent that helps reduce nervous tension. It is a traditional Chinese and Indian medicinal and culinary plant that has a stimulating effect on the whole system.

To revive your spirits or combat lethargy while you work, put a few drops in an aromatherapy burner. Before a big night out, add a few drops to your bath, and revel in its head-clearing aroma.

Lemongrass is cleansing and astringent and makes an excellent deodorant, especially if you perspire excessively. It tightens and refines a lackluster skin, so it makes a good toning lotion and works well in steam inhalation. A few drops of lemongrass on your hairbrush will revive lank hair. Use in a foot bath to refresh sweaty feet.

*Caution: May be irritating to sensitive skin. Avoid during pregnancy.*

**Lime** *(Citrus acris or Citrus aurantifolia)* • **Fruit** • **Top Note**

The refreshing, uplifting scent of lime will heighten the joy of a happy relationship, adding a sense of playfulness. Lime will help clear the mind and ease the anxieties that can provoke problems in relationships. Use it in a bath or aromatherapy burner.

As a skin-care oil, lime's citrusy tang is of particular benefit to oily skin. Use it as an ingredient in men's aftershave. It is also wonderful for use in a foot bath, especially on hot, humid days.

Essential oil of lime is also useful in a blend for the temporary relief of catarrh, sinusitis, and chest infections. Use it in a steam inhalation, an aromatherapy burner, a bath, or massage-oil blend. *Caution: May be irritating to sensitive skin and may increase photosensitivity. Do not use before exposure to the sun.*

**Neroli** *(Citrus aurantium or Citrus vulgaris)* • **Flower** • **Middle to Base Note**

One of the most expensive of the oils, it takes one ton of flowers to yield 2 pounds (1 kg) of oil, so it is usually sold 3 percent in jojoba oil. Neroli, also known as orange flower oil, was used in the first eau de Cologne in the 18th century.

Neroli is a slightly hypnotic oil that reduces anxiety. While neroli is beneficial in all kinds of stressful situations, it is especially useful for reducing the anxiety associated with sexual relationships, as the scent is sensual and encourages romantic feelings. Use it in a bath, a massage-oil blend, or dab a few drops on your pillow. Oils blended with jojoba are not suitable for burning.

Use it in a skin-oil blend with geranium and frankincense for dry, sensitive, and mature skin.

**Orange** *(Citrus aurantium or Citrus vulgaris)* • **Fruit Rind** • **Top Note**

Like the other citrus oils, orange brings warmth and cheer to uplift the spirits and calm the nerves. Its light-hearted sensuousness is beneficial to those suffering from depression or a lack of energy, and to relationships that have drifted into routine and repetition. Use in an aromatherapy burner to create a jubilant atmosphere, add a few drops to your bath, or add to a massage-oil blend.

Orange is useful in a skin-oil blend for dry or mature skin. The skin-oil blend is also a useful treatment for eczema. Orange brings temporary relief from insomnia, coughs, colds, and flu.

*Caution: May irritate sensitive skins and may increase skin photosensitivity. Do not use prior to exposure to the sun.*

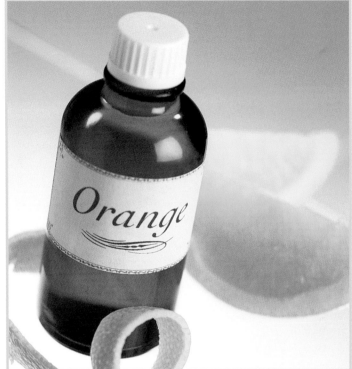

## Patchouli
### (Pogostemon patchouli) •
### Leaf • Base Note

This is the scent the hippies of the '60s and '70s embraced to promote love and peace, but this rich, exotic scent is one you will either love or hate. Patchouli is believed to be an aphrodisiac, especially when blended with ylang-ylang, and it has been widely used in love potions.

It is also an oil that is used in meditation, especially when combined with sandalwood and frankincense. Patchouli will decrease inhibition and increase the ability to communicate. It is effective in treating anxiety and depression and is deeply relaxing.

When blended in a skin oil, patchouli is a good skin-care treatment for dry and mature skin. It is warming, so it is an excellent choice for cold weather.

## Peppermint *(Mentha piperita)* • Herb • Top Note

Peppermint stimulates the brain and promotes clear thinking. It revives you when you are emotionally or physically exhausted — just inhale from the bottle for an immediate lift.

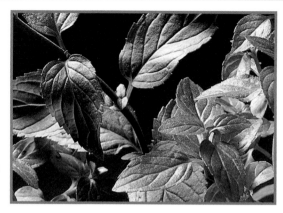

An excellent remedy for nausea and hangover, it cools fever and settles the stomach. Make peppermint part of your travel kit: It is an excellent remedy for travel sickness and jetlag. Use in an aromatherapy burner, or for direct inhalation and steam inhalation, or take 1 drop in a glass of water.

The invigorating flavor of peppermint makes it a refreshing mouthwash. Add 1 drop to half a glass of water. A drop added to your shampoo or hair conditioner will stimulate the scalp.

Peppermint is also effective in bringing relief from headaches, colds, flu, sinusitis, and congestion.

*Caution: Do not use during pregnancy.*

## Petitgrain *(Citrus aurantium)* • Leaf and Twig • Top to Middle Note

Steam-distilled from the leaves, twigs and unripe baby oranges of the tree, this oil is also known as "poor man's neroli." Like neroli, petitgrain is an ingredient in several perfumes and colognes.

Petitgrain has clarifying and uplifting properties and relieves restlessness, mild anxiety, tension, and stress. Use a few drops on a compress to calm nervous, perspiring bodies. A few drops in your bath or massage-oil blend has a wonderfully uplifting effect.

A few drops of this astringent essence in your facial oil has a healing effect on blemished skin. Use in a direct application for acne. Put it in a final rinse for oily hair. Used in a deodorant, petitgrain will help reduce excessive perspiration.

*Caution: May be irritating to sensitive skin and may increase skin photosensitivity. Do not use prior to exposure to the sun.*

## Rose *(Rosa centifolia/damascena/gallica)*
## • Flower • Middle to Base Note

The red petals of 30 blooms are needed to produce just 1 drop of rose oil. The most expensive of all the oils, it is usually sold as a 3 percent distilled essential oil in a jojoba oil base. Oils in a jojoba oil base are not suitable for use in an oil burner.

Roses have been celebrated in myth and legend as the flower of seduction and in all matters of love. Rose essential oil also has a positive effect on sexual problems, as it is soothing to the nerves, healing to the heart, and helps disperse fear and negativity. Use in a bath, as a personal perfume, or in a massage-oil blend.

Rose used in a facial-oil blend has a restorative effect on all skin types, especially mature skin.

## Rosemary *(Rosmarinus officinalis)*
## • Herb • Middle Note

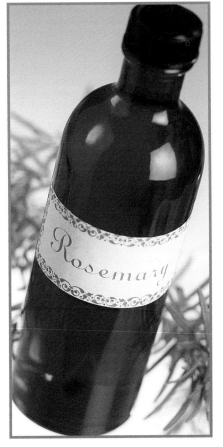

Brisk, clear, and penetrating are the words usually used to describe this oil. Rosemary oil energizes mental activity, revitalizes memory, and aids concentration, so it is an excellent oil to use in an aromatherapy burner while you are studying for exams or working at any task that requires concentration.

For headaches or for an immediate lift, apply directly to the forehead and temples. A bath or a massage using a rosemary oil blend will also help revive and revitalize you.

Rosemary makes a wonderful hair tonic. Just add it to the final rinse water or sprinkle it on your hairbrush. Direct inhalation from the bottle or 5 drops in an aromatherapy burner will ease morning sickness — however, do not use in any other way during pregnancy.

*Caution: Not to be used by persons suffering from epilepsy or high blood pressure.*

## Rosewood *(Aniba rosaeodora)* • **Wood** • **Top to Middle Note**

Its warm, rich, spicy scent is extremely balancing and calming when you are under stress. It has an uplifting and reassuring quality that enables you to press forward despite difficulties.

These qualities make rosewood oil an invaluable aid in helping you to resolve issues with your partner or to calm a supersensitive nature. Use it in an aromatherapy burner, a bath, or a massage-oil blend. When events seems to be getting too much to handle, use it as a direct application to the temples, massaging gently.

Rosewood is an excellent remedy for the strains of long-distance traveling. Keep a bottle as part of your travel kit.

Used in a facial oil, rosewood balances skin problems. Use it as a direct application for cold sores, acne, and dermatitis. Its antibacterial and antiseptic properties make rosewood a good deodorant. Its warm, woody scent makes a delightful aftershave.

## Sage *(Salvia officinalis)* • **Leaf**

Sage has a mellow, musky scent and has an astringent, cooling effect. It acts to cleanse and calm both the mind and the skin.

The ancient Greeks believed sage extended their life spans, while the Egyptians used it to increase their fertility. Nowadays, sage is used in the treatment of premenstrual syndrome and some symptoms of menopause.

Its calming properties seem to have a positive effect in countering frigidity, as well as in helping to ease nervous tension. Use in an aromatherapy burner, in a bath, or in a massage-oil blend. It is also an effective remedy for rheumatism and muscular aches and pains.

Sage is an extremely effective deodorant and antiperspirant. It can also be used diluted in distilled water as a gargle and mouthwash.

*Caution: Avoid use during pregnancy.*

## Sandalwood *(Santalum album)* • Wood • Base Note

Loved by both men and women, sandalwood is one of the most sensually stirring of the essential oils. It contains a constituent that resembles androsterone, a male pheromone. Sandalwood oil is distilled from the heart of the sandalwood tree, which grows in Mysore, India, and is not harvested until it has reached the end of its life.

Sandalwood has been used in Indian spiritual and sexual practices for centuries. Its aroma encourages communication and an opening up of your inner being. Its nurturing, stabilizing, and strengthening effect on the emotions may assist you in letting go of fears and phobias that may be preventing you from making the most out of your life.

Used in a facial oil, sandalwood is beneficial for dry and mature skins. It makes an excellent aftershave.

## Ylang-Ylang *(Cananga odorata)* • Flower • Middle to Base Note

Known in the Philippines as the flower of flowers, the blossoms of ylang-ylang are spread over the beds of newlyweds. Because its scent is sweet, intoxicating, exotic, and erotic, ylang-ylang is often used in perfumes — including Chanel No. 5.

Ylang-ylang is soothing to feelings of anger, jealousy, panic, and fear. It calms anxiety and overstimulation, while boosting low energy. Ylang-ylang has a sedative effect and is useful at times of high levels of stress. It is also an effective treatment for insomnia.

This oil has a balancing effect on skin that is either too dry or too oily. A few drops added to shampoo or conditioner will stimulate healthy hair growth.

*Caution: Excessive use may cause nausea and headache.*

# Compatible Oils

**Basil:** Black pepper, bergamot, all citrus essential oils, geranium, lavender, marjoram, neroli, petitgrain, peppermint, rosemary

**Bergamot:** All citrus essential oils, and most other oils

**Black pepper:** Basil, bergamot, cypress, frankincense, geranium, ginger, grapefruit, lavender, lemon, marjoram, palmarosa, rosemary, sandalwood, ylang-ylang

**Calendula (macerated oil):** Cypress, lemon, myrrh

**Cedarwood:** Bergamot, all citrus oils, cypress, eucalyptus, geranium, jasmine, juniper, lavender, neroli, petitgrain, rose, rosewood, rosemary, sandalwood, ylang-ylang

**Chamomile:** Bergamot, all citrus oils, cypress, geranium, lavender, jasmine, marjoram, neroli, petitgrain, rosewood, sandalwood, vetiver, ylang-ylang

**Clary sage:** Cypress, geranium, grapefruit, jasmine, lavender, lemon, neroli, orange, patchouli, petitgrain, rose, sage, sandalwood, ylang-ylang

**Cypress:** Bergamot, cedarwood, chamomile, all citrus oils, clary sage, geranium, juniper, lavender, marjoram, pine, rose, rosewood, rosemary, sandalwood

**Frankincense:** Basil, bergamot, black pepper, all citrus oils, geranium, jasmine, lavender, lemongrass, myrrh, neroli, pine, rose, rosewood, petitgrain, rose, patchouli, sandalwood, vetiver, ylang-ylang

**Geranium:** Basil, bergamot, all citrus oils, clary sage, cypress, frankincense, juniper, lavender, marjoram, neroli, rose, rosewood, sandalwood, ylang-ylang

**Ginger:** Black pepper, bergamot, cedarwood, geranium, jasmine, lemon, marjoram, neroli, orange, patchouli, rose, rosewood, rosemary, sandalwood, ylang-ylang

**Grapefruit:** Basil, bergamot, chamomile, all citrus essential oils, clary sage, cypress, eucalyptus, frankincense, geranium, juniper, lavender, lemongrass, myrrh, marjoram, palmarosa, peppermint, petitgrain, rosemary

**Jasmine:** Bergamot, clary sage, frankincense, grapefruit, lavender, rose, rosewood, sandalwood, ylang-ylang

**Juniper:** Bergamot, all citrus oils, cypress, geranium, lavender, neroli, petitgrain, rose, rosemary, rosewood, sandalwood

**Lavender:** All essential oils — especially bergamot, clary sage, geranium, marjoram, lemon, neroli, orange, petitgrain, rose, rosemary, ylang-ylang

**Lemon:** Basil, bergamot, black pepper, cedarwood, chamomile, all citrus oils, clary sage, cypress, frankincense, geranium, juniper, lavender, neroli, patchouli, petitgrain, rose, rosemary, sandalwood

**Lemongrass:** Bergamot, black pepper, cedarwood, all citrus oils, cypress, frankincense, geranium, jasmine, juniper, lavender, neroli, rose, rosemary, rosewood, tea tree

**Lime:** Bergamot, all citrus oils, lavender

**Neroli:** Calendula, chamomile, all citrus oils, clary sage, frankincense, geranium, jasmine, lavender, marjoram, myrrh, patchouli, petitgrain, rose, rosewood, sandalwood, vetiver, ylang-ylang

**Orange, Sweet:** Bergamot, clary sage, all citrus oils, cypress, frankincense, geranium, jasmine, juniper, lavender, neroli, petitgrain, rose, rosewood, sandalwood, ylang-ylang

**Patchouli:** Bergamot, all citrus oils, chamomile, clary sage, cypress, frankincense, geranium, lavender, myrrh, neroli, rose, rosewood, sandalwood, vetiver, ylang-ylang

**Peppermint:** Basil, bergamot, black pepper, cedarwood, all citrus oils, cypress, eucalyptus, juniper, lavender, marjoram, rosemary

**Petitgrain:** Bergamot, black pepper, cedarwood, chamomile, all citrus oils, clary sage, cypress, frankincense, geranium, jasmine, juniper, lavender, marjoram, myrrh, neroli, rose, rosemary, peppermint, sandalwood, ylang-ylang

**Rose:** Bergamot, chamomile, all citrus oils, clary sage, cypress, frankincense, geranium, jasmine, lavender, marjoram, myrrh, neroli, patchouli, peppermint, petitgrain, orange, rosemary, rosewood, sandalwood, ylang-ylang

**Rosemary:** Basil, bergamot, black pepper, chamomile, all citrus oils, cypress, frankincense, geranium, ginger, jasmine, juniper, lavender, lemongrass, marjoram, neroli, petitgrain, rosewood, sandalwood, ylang-ylang

**Rosewood:** Bergamot, cedarwood, frankincense, geranium, lavender, neroli, orange, palmarosa, patchouli, petitgrain, rose, rosemary, sandalwood, ylang-ylang

**Sage:** Bergamot, cedarwood, clary sage, jasmine, juniper, lavender, orange, rosemary, sandalwood

**Sandalwood:** Benzoin, bergamot, chamomile, all citrus oils, clary sage, frankincense, geranium, jasmine, lavender, marjoram, myrrh, neroli, patchouli, petitgrain, rose, rosemary, sage, vetiver, ylang-ylang

**Ylang-Ylang:** Benzoin, bergamot, chamomile, all citrus oils, clary sage, cypress, frankincense, geranium, jasmine, marjoram, myrrh, neroli, patchouli, petitgrain, rose, rosewood, sandalwood, vetiver

# Oils and Their Effects

## On the Emotions and the Senses

| THE OIL | Opens Love | Heightens Sensuality | Erotic | Uplifts Spirits | Calms Anxiety | Courage & Strength | Balances Emotions | Harmony & Unity | Clarity of Mind | Comfort |
|---|---|---|---|---|---|---|---|---|---|---|
| Basil | | ◉ | ◉ | ◉ | ◉ | | | | | |
| Bergamot | | ◉ | | ◉ | ◉ | | ◉ | | ◉ | ◉ |
| Black Pepper | ◉ | ◉ | ◉ | | | ◉ | | | ◉ | |
| Calendula | | | | | ◉ | | | ◉ | | ◉ |
| Cedarwood | ◉ | ◉ | | | ◉ | | | ◉ | | ◉ |
| Chamomile | | | | | ◉ | | ◉ | | | |
| Clary Sage | ◉ | ◉ | ◉ | ◉ | | | ◉ | ◉ | | |
| Frankincense | ◉ | ◉ | | ◉ | ◉ | | ◉ | ◉ | | ◉ |
| Geranium | | ◉ | | ◉ | ◉ | | ◉◉ | | | |
| Ginger | | ◉ | ◉ | ◉ | | | | | | |
| Jasmine | ◉ | ◉ | ◉ | ◉ | | ◉ | | | | ◉ |
| Juniper | ◉ | ◉ | ◉ | | ◉ | ◉ | ◉ | ◉ | ◉ | |
| Lavender | ◉ | ◉ | | ◉ | ◉ | ◉ | ◉ | ◉ | | ◉ |
| Lemon | | ◉ | | ◉ | ◉ | | | | ◉ | |
| Lemongrass | | ◉ | | | | | | | ◉ | |
| Lime | | ◉ | | ◉ | | | | | | |
| Marjoram | | | | | | | | | | ◉ |
| Myrrh | | | | | | ◉ | | | | |
| Neroli | ◉ | ◉ | ◉ | ◉ | ◉ | | | ◉ | | |
| Orange | | ◉ | | ◉ | ◉ | | | | | |
| Patchouli | ◉ | ◉ | ◉ | ◉ | ◉ | | | ◉ | | |
| Peppermint | | | | ◉ | | | | | ◉ | |
| Petitgrain | | | | ◉ | ◉ | | | | | |
| Rose | ◉ | ◉ | ◉ | ◉ | ◉ | | ◉ | ◉ | | ◉ |
| Rosemary | | | | ◉ | | | | | ◉ | |
| Rosewood | | | | | ◉ | | ◉ | | ◉ | |
| Sage | | | | | ◉ | | ◉ | | ◉ | |
| Sandalwood | ◉ | ◉ | ◉ | ◉ | ◉ | ◉ | ◉ | ◉ | | ◉ |
| Vetiver | | | | | ◉ | | ◉ | ◉ | | ◉ |
| Ylang-Ylang | ◉ | ◉ | ◉ | ◉ | ◉ | | ◉ | ◉ | | ◉ |

# Skin Care

| THE OIL | Dry Skin | Mature Skin | Oily Skin | Sensitive Skin | Acne | Special | Mouth-wash | Deod-orant | Feet | Hair | After-shave |
|---|---|---|---|---|---|---|---|---|---|---|---|
| Bergamot | | | ◎ | ◎ | ◎ | E, D | ◎ | | | | |
| Calendula | ◎ | ◎ | | ◎ | | CS | | | | | |
| Cedarwood | ◎ | ◎ | ◎ | | ◎ | IS | | | | ◎ | ◎ |
| Chamomile | ◎ | | ◎ | ◎ | ◎ | E, BC | | | | ◎ | |
| Cypress | | ◎ | ◎ | | | E, BC | | ◎ | ◎ | | ◎ |
| Frankincense | | ◎ | ◎ | | | E, BC | | | | | |
| Geranium | ◎ | ◎ | ◎ | ◎ | ◎ | E, BC | | | ◎ | | |
| Jasmine | ◎ | ◎ | ◎ | ◎ | | | | | | ◎ | |
| Juniper | | | ◎ | | ◎ | E | | | | ◎ | ◎ |
| Lavender | ◎ | | ◎ | ◎ | ◎ | E | | | | | |
| Lemon | ◎ | | ◎ | | ◎ | DS | ◎ | ◎ | ◎ | ◎ | |
| Lemongrass | | | | | ◎ | DS | | ◎ | ◎ | ◎ | |
| Lime | | | | | | | | ◎ | ◎ | | ◎ |
| Marjoram | | | | | | | | | ◎ | ◎ | ◎ |
| Myrrh | | | | | | | ◎ | | | | |
| Neroli | ◎ | ◎ | | ◎ | | | | | | | |
| Orange | ◎ | ◎ | ◎ | ◎ | | E | ◎ | | | | |
| Patchouli | ◎ | ◎ | ◎ | | ◎ | | | | ◎ | ◎ | |
| Palmarosa | | ◎ | ◎ | | ◎ | D | | | | | |
| Peppermint | | | ◎ | | | | ◎ | | ◎ | ◎ | |
| Petitgrain | | | ◎ | | ◎ | B | | ◎ | ◎ | ◎ | |
| Pine | | | | | | | | ◎ | ◎ | | |
| Rose | ◎ | ◎ | ◎ | ◎ | | BC | | | | | ◎ |
| Rosemary | | | ◎ | | | | | | ◎ | ◎ | |
| Rosewood | ◎ | ◎ | ◎ | | ◎ | D | | ◎ | ◎ | ◎ | ◎ |
| Sage | | | | | | | ◎ | ◎ | ◎ | | |
| Sandalwood | ◎ | ◎ | | ◎ | ◎ | E | | | | ◎ | ◎ |
| Thyme | | | | | | | | | ◎ | | |
| Vetiver | | | ◎ | | ◎ | | | | | | ◎ |
| Ylang-Ylang | ◎ | | ◎ | | | | | | | ◎ | |

B: Blemishes;  BC: Broken Capillaries;  CS: Chapped Skin;  D: Dermatitis;  DS: Dull Skin;
E: Eczema;  IS: Inflamed Skin

# Music for Massage and Aromatherapy

*Truly fertile Music, the only kind that will move us, that we shall truly appreciate, will be a Music conducive to Dream, which banishes all reason and analysis. One must not wish first to understand and then to feel. Art does not tolerate Reason.*

**Albert Camus,** *Youthful Writings*

Music, like scent, can open your senses and loosen the grip of your mind and intellect. The following selection has been chosen for the soothing rhythms and beautiful melodies, which are sure to enhance your massage, aromabath, or any other enjoyment of simple pleasures.

## Voice

*Kyrie* by Palestrina

*Miserere mei, Deus* by Allegri

Lieder by Schubert, Mendelssohn, Schumann, Wolf

*Songs of the Auverne* by Cantaloube

*Cantique de Jean Racine* by Fauré

Songs by Grieg, Franck, Fauré

*Agnes Dei* by Samuel Barber

## Strings

Canon in D by Pachelbel

Adagio in G minor by Albinoni

*The Four Seasons* by Vivaldi

*Brandenberg Concertos* by J.S. Bach

Sonatas for Violin and Keyboard by J.S. Bach

Sonatas for Viola da Gamba and Keyboard by J.S. Bach

Piano Quintet in A, Op. 114 by Schubert ("Trout")

String Quartet No. 12 in F, Op. 96 by Dvorak ("American")

*Adagio for Strings* by Samuel Barber

## Orchestra

*Water Music* by Handel

*Pastoral Symphony* by Beethoven

*La Mer* by Debussy

*Daphnis et Chloe* Suite No. 2 by Ravel

*Pavane for a Dead Princess* by Ravel

*Fantasia on a Theme of Thomas Tallis* by
Vaughan Williams

*The Lark Ascending* by Vaughan Williams

## Other Instruments

Oboe Concerto in D minor, Op. 9 No. 2 by
Albinoni

Suite in A minor for Recorder and Strings by
Telemann

Clarinet Concerto in A by Mozart

Flute Concerto No. 1 in G by Mozart

Arrangements for flute and harp of pieces by
Debussy, Ravel, Fauré, and others

## Piano

*Goldberg Variations* by J.S. Bach

Piano Concertos Nos. 20, 21, 23, 24 by Mozart

Piano Concerto in A minor, Op. 85 by Hummel

Waltzes by Chopin

Nocturnes by Chopin

*Songs Without Words* by Mendelssohn

*Scenes from Childhood* by Schumann

*Children's Corner* by Debussy

*Sonatine* by Ravel

*Pavane for a Dead Princess* by Ravel

# Aromatic Beauty Treatments

As we age, our skins lose elasticity and the freshness of youth. Essential oils are packed with nutrients and proteins that help to maintain the collagen responsible for that fresh, firm appearance. They promote blood circulation and stimulate the lymphatic system, which is responsible for removing toxins from the body. In addition, essential oils have such beautiful scents that they will turn your daily skin care routine into a luxurious ritual.

Following are some simple beauty treatments you can make at home using essential oils.

## Basic Requirements

• Sterilized, dark glass jars and bottles for storing creams and toners • Bowls for mixing • Beeswax • Honey • Yogurt • Fruit • Oatmeal, cornmeal, ground almonds, or ground hazelnuts • Cider vinegar • Vodka • Purified water • Essential oils to suit your skin type

## Cleansers

There are several choices when deciding what type of cleanser to use. You can use vegetable soaps or special cleansing bars and water; you can use creams that you have either purchased or made yourself (see page 76); or you can use simple vegetable oils enhanced with essential oils.

All vegetable and nut oils can be used for cleansing and nourishing the skin. Add 4 to 6 drops of up to three essential oils for your skin type (see chart on page 69) to every 2 tablespoons (30 ml) carrier oil in a dark glass bottle with a dropper. Shake well before use and massage into your skin. If using as a cleanser, scrape off oil with a tissue or with cotton pads soaked in toner. Rinse your face thoroughly with tepid water or toner, and moisturize.

Essential oils with good cleansing properties and suitable for all skin types are chamomile, clary sage, geranium, lavender, lemon, lime, sage, and thyme. Rosemary is good for oily skin.

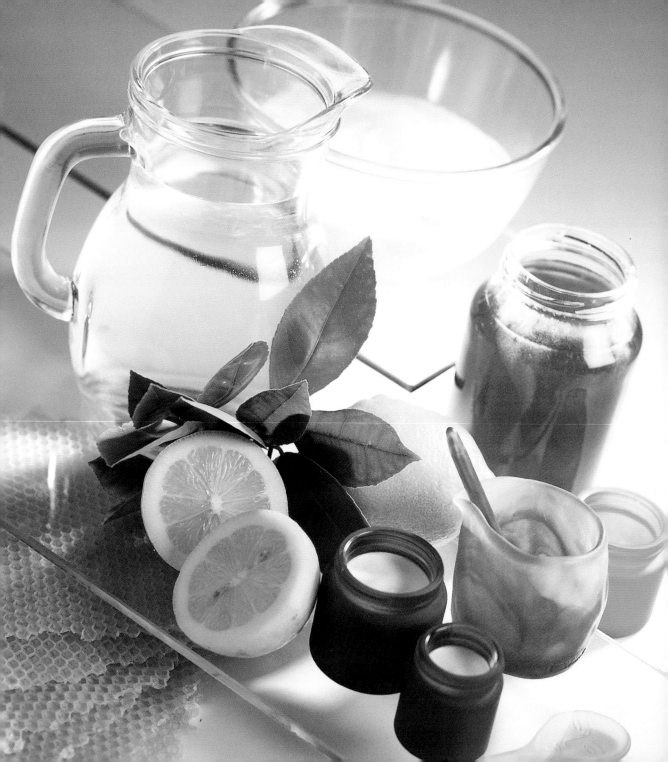

# Facial Scrubs and Masks

Use a facial mask or scrub once or twice a week, or whenever your skin feels a little rough. It will stimulate the skin and blood circulation and exfoliate the dead cells that inhibit moisturizing and give your skin that dull look.

**Cereals and nuts**— oatmeal, cornmeal, almonds, and hazelnuts — make excellent scrubs.

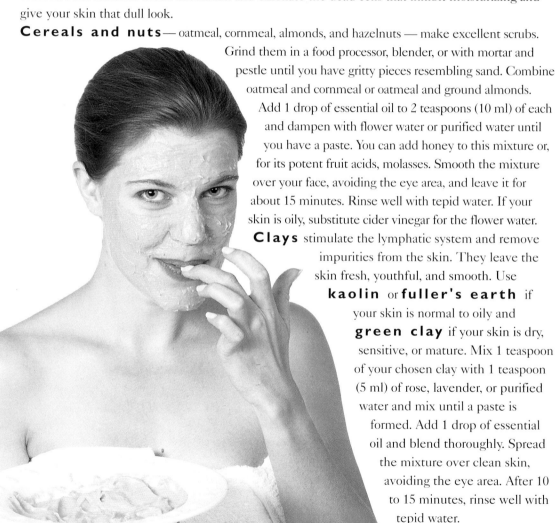

Grind them in a food processor, blender, or with mortar and pestle until you have gritty pieces resembling sand. Combine oatmeal and cornmeal or oatmeal and ground almonds. Add 1 drop of essential oil to 2 teaspoons (10 ml) of each and dampen with flower water or purified water until you have a paste. You can add honey to this mixture or, for its potent fruit acids, molasses. Smooth the mixture over your face, avoiding the eye area, and leave it for about 15 minutes. Rinse well with tepid water. If your skin is oily, substitute cider vinegar for the flower water.

**Clays** stimulate the lymphatic system and remove impurities from the skin. They leave the skin fresh, youthful, and smooth. Use **kaolin** or **fuller's earth** if your skin is normal to oily and **green clay** if your skin is dry, sensitive, or mature. Mix 1 teaspoon of your chosen clay with 1 teaspoon (5 ml) of rose, lavender, or purified water and mix until a paste is formed. Add 1 drop of essential oil and blend thoroughly. Spread the mixture over clean skin, avoiding the eye area. After 10 to 15 minutes, rinse well with tepid water.

**Fruit and yogurt** make excellent masks. Mash 1 tablespoon of pawpaw or avocado or take 1 tablespoon (15 ml) of yogurt and add 1 drop of essential oil. Mix well. Apply to clean skin, avoiding the eye area. After 10 to15 minutes, rinse well with tepid water.

**Molasses** makes an excellent scrub or mask because it is a rich source of alpha hydroxy acids (A.H.A.), which are mild acids from plants that perform an exfoliating function. Just smear it on while you are in the bath or shower (it is very messy but feels great), massage in, and leave on for up to 15 minutes. Rinse off with clean, tepid water; your skin will feel smooth and vibrant. Most of the best cosmetic companies are promoting very expensive creams containing A.H.A. Why pay all that money when you can buy a large bottle of molasses for a fraction of the cost?

## Toners

Toners make your skin feel fresh and alive. They help close the pores and should be used after cleansing. You can apply toner by soaking cotton pads and wiping them over your face and neck in upward strokes, or you can splash it on.

If your skin is **dry**, **mature**, or **sensitive**, do not use an astringent or toner containing alcohol. Rose or lavender water on its own makes a wonderful toner or you can add 10 drops of up to two essential oils to every 7 tablespoons (100 ml) purified water or 5 tablespoons (70 ml) purified water and 2 tablespoons (30 ml) glycerin. Shake the bottle thoroughly before each use.

You can make your own flower water by adding 10 drops of your favorite essential oil to 7 tablespoons (100 ml) purified water. Always shake thoroughly before use. Rose, lavender, and orange (including neroli and petitgrain) make wonderful flower waters. If using rose, jasmine, or neroli essential oil that has been blended in jojoba oil, you will need to mix it with a solubalizer *before* adding it to the water.

If your skin is **oily**, use up to 4 teaspoons (20 ml) vodka or cider vinegar to 5 tablespoons (80 ml) purified water. Add 10 drops of up to three essential oils and shake thoroughly before use. Witch hazel is another suitable ingredient to use in a toner for people with oily skin. Use 2 tablespoons (30 ml) of witch hazel to 5 tablespoons (70 ml) purified water or flower water and shake thoroughly before use.

# *Moisturizing Creams*

Apply moisturizing creams to your skin after cleansing and toning. Make sure your skin is moist before you apply cream. Dab spots of cream at various points over your face and neck, and then, with the pads of your fingers, massage the cream into your skin, using small circular motions that move upward and outward. Do not forget your neck and chest area. These require the same amount of attention you give to your face. Gently press the cream into the eye area; the skin here is very delicate. After massaging, lightly slap your face and neck all over with the pads of your fingers. This will energize both you and your skin.

*Never apply cream to dry skin. It will pull the skin, causing sagging and wrinkling.*

| Dry-to-Normal Skin | Normal-to-Oily Skin | Sensitive Skin |
|---|---|---|
| 1 tablespoon shaved beeswax | 1 tablespoon shaved beeswax | 1 tablespoon shaved beeswax |
| 5 teaspoons (25 ml) jojoba oil | 3 teaspoons (15 ml) jojoba oil | 4 tablespoons (60 ml) sweet almond oil |
| 3 teaspoons (15 ml) avocado oil | 5 teaspoons (25 ml) grapeseed oil | 8 teaspoons (40 ml) purified water |
| 5 teaspoons (25 ml) sweet almond oil | 5 teaspoons (25 ml) cider vinegar | *4 to 6 drops rose essential oil |
| 5 teaspoons (25 ml) purified water | 4 teaspoons (20 ml) purified water | |
| 4 to 6 drops essential oils | 4 to 6 drops essential oils | |

You can buy solid blocks of beeswax from health food stores. Shave off flakes with a knife or vegetable peeler. Melt the beeswax over a very low heat and stir in the oils. Keep stirring until oils and beeswax are completely melted. Slowly add the water and keep stirring until beeswax, oils, and water are properly blended. Take the pot off the heat. Add the essential oils while stirring constantly. Mix well using an electric whisk or blender until the mixture is cool. Store in a sterilized, dark glass jar.

If you like, you can add a teaspoon of honey or honeycomb to the beeswax. This will make the cream richer and thicker. You can also alter the consistency by using slightly more or less beeswax.

* Variation for sensitive skin: You may prefer jasmine, geranium, lavender, or neroli essentil oil.

## Deodorant

Pour 5 tablespoons (80 ml) vodka and
4 teaspoons (20 ml) purified water into a
4-ounce (100 ml) dark glass bottle or spray
container and shake vigorously to mix
contents.

Blend together in a glass container or on a spoon:

5 drops sage

5 drops lemon

5 drops lemongrass

OR

5 drops juniper

5 drops petitgrain

5 drops lemongrass

OR

A combination of your own oils listed in the
chart on page 69.

Add this blend to the vodka and purified
water. Shake thoroughly to mix all the
ingredients.

*Note: Quantities can be altered to suit your needs.*

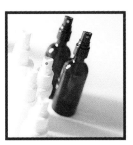

## Aftershave

If your skin is dry or sensitive, do not use an
aftershave containing alcohol. A moisturizing
oil blend will invigorate your skin and leave it
feeling soft and smooth.

Blend together in a glass container or on a spoon:

5 drops of sage

5 drops cedarwood

5 drops juniper

OR

5 drops sandalwood

5 drops petitgrain

5 drops marjoram

OR

15 drops of up to 3 oils of your choice
from the chart on page 69.

Add this blend to 7 tablespoons (100 ml)
sweet almond oil in a dark glass bottle and
shake thoroughly.

If you would prefer that alcoholic zing, put
5 tablespoons (80 ml) vodka and 4 teaspoons
(20 ml) purified water into a 4-ounce (100 ml)
bottle and add the essential oil blend.
Shake thoroughly.

# Index

Copyright © Lansdowne Publishing Pty Ltd
First published 1997

TIME-LIFE BOOKS IS A DIVISION OF TIME LIFE INC.

TIME-LIFE CUSTOM PUBLISHING

| | |
|---|---|
| Vice President and Publisher | Terry Newell |
| Associate Publisher | Teresa Hartnett |
| Vice President of Sales and Marketing | Neil Levin |
| Director of New Product Development | Quentin McAndrew |
| Director of Special Sales | Liz Ziehl |
| Project Manager | Teresa Graham |

TIME-LIFE is a trademark of Time Warner Inc. U.S.A.

ISBN 0-7835-5256-4
CIP data available upon application:
Librarian
Time-Life Books
2000 Duke Street
Alexandria, VA 22314

Printed in Singapore by Tien Wah Press (Pte) Ltd

Quotes on pages 8 and 70 from *The Columbia Dictionary of Quotations*.
Translations on pages 46 and 47 from *Daughters of Isis*, J. Tyldesley, London: Penguin, 1995.